LAST ONE HOME

SHARI J. RYAN

Heather ♡
Thank you for
all of your support!
I hope you enjoy!
xoxo
Sha~

Shari J Ryan
USA TODAY BESTSELLING AUTHOR

LAST ONE HOME

SHARI J. RYAN

Copyright © 2021 by Shari J. Ryan
ISBN: **978-1-7363876-1-0**
LCCN: 2020925642

Edited by Cindy Dimpfl

To my grandparents, Marcia and Al—
For being the inspiration of eternal love, devotion, and purpose.

"You must do the thing you think you cannot do."

— ELEANOR ROOSEVELT

PROLOGUE
JULY 2017

SWIRLS OF OIL, like the feathers of a peacock, in hues of blue, green, and turquoise memorialize a moment in time.

Pearl's tranquil, warm water ripples around my feet as I revere in the horizon's beauty—the thin line that separates the ocean and sky, rendering a mirrored reflection from one side to the other.

I close my eyes, welcoming the Hawaiian warmth to penetrate my skin, and my mind drifts out to sea, recalling the day, which President Roosevelt warned, would live in infamy.

Any source of clean air is sparse as black clouds of smoke bloom in every direction, and the world shatters beneath me.

The hum and whistles of explosives raining down from the sky are striking recollections of a nightmare that will never fade. Like film spinning on its reel until there was nothing left to view, I stood there still as a statue, frozen in time, with only seconds to ponder my options: to run away or step into the fire.

There were so many lives to save, but all I could see at that moment were arms, waving and pleading from the sloshing waters as their bodies incinerated. They were boys; young men who sacrificed their futures to protect our country and shouldn't have had to die on American territory.

I couldn't ignore the screams, cries, and pleas for help, and I questioned if I was the only one who could assist. My life was in jeopardy, like theirs, but I wanted to save as many as I could. For some, that meant merely holding a hand as they took their final breaths. Nothing could be worse than dying alone, and I knew offering comfort in their last moments was more important than saving myself.

I have lived a lifetime since this tragic day, wondering if I could have done more, but just as we can't predict the future, it's impossible to change the past.

Now, I'm left to wonder how far I must travel to find *my* way home. I don't know whether the waters will carry me gently to familiar shores or if the currents would pull me away, out to the white cap peaks beyond the clear blue water.

"It's already been such a long, fulfilling journey, but it was always meant to be with you," I speak into the wind. "I miss you terribly, darling, and like Frank Sinatra said, *'I'm afraid I'll never smile again until I smile at you ...'*"

This is where my life began, and where it shall end.

1

CURRENT DAY - OCTOBER 2018

MY APRICOT-COLORED CHAISE LOUNGE, two matching guest chairs, and a small mango wood stand are all the furniture I need on this terrace.

Years ago, we had all the outdoor-living accoutrements. With a brick oven and grill, a stone centerpiece made up of sea glass, and several spots to sit at a weathered picnic-table, we had plenty of space to fit our large family. The sides of my tongue tingle just thinking about the sweetness of grilled pineapple. There was something special about the cool tangy taste among a humid night embodied by the whisking scent of rich botanicals and salty Pacific mist.

It has certainly been a while since I've hosted a dinner here, but I prefer simplicity these days. Plus, with the abundance of potted greenery and the sheer walls designed for a full view of the ocean, I'm complacent most of the time. At least, I presume to be. Not everyone can say they look in a mirror and find an unfamiliar person staring back at them, but I suppose this is just another one of life's mysteries.

The low roar of a car's engine crawls along the winding driveway to the left of my chair. I don't believe I'm expecting company, but an invitation to my residence has never been necessary. In fact, I enjoy surprise visits.

I bend forward and take hold of the armrest for support while seeking a glimpse of the car. A sharp, sporty black sedan parks along the left side of the driveway, but I don't recognize the vehicle or the well-dressed man stepping out onto the pavement.

Keiki, my live-in caretaker, will handle whatever the man needs. She's the sole reason I can continue to live in the luxury of what we once built as a forever home. If it wasn't for her, the upkeep of the house would be far too much work to take on alone. And I refuse to burden my family with such nonsense.

I release my hold against the armrests and lean back into my chair as the shine of a red ribbon catches my eye. I don't recall bringing the new notebook outside with me, but maybe Keiki left it on the table in case I wanted to make some notes. My granddaughter—Makena, she was such a sweetheart to gift me the book. It even has my name etched into the leather. I open the pages to the ribbon marked spot, but there aren't any reminders about appointments or visitors today. I suppose the gentleman must be a tourist trying to find his way downtown, but knowing Keiki, she will gather a notepaper and a pen from her pocket and write out precise directions for the poor man.

A faint knock on the outside of the room draws my attention through the open glass fixtures. "Yes," I call out. "Keiki, is that you?"

The bedroom door swooshes open just wide enough for Keiki to poke her head in. Her long, silky dark hair falls to the side of her shoulders and her teeth glow against the coral pink coloring of her lips. With eyes that can tell hundreds of stories before speaking a single word, she appears perplexed.

"Good morning, honey. You have an unexpected visitor. I also have your breakfast if you're ready." Her voice is serene and dainty, but also clear and crisp. Keiki worked at a rejuvenation spa before coming to care for me. She has the patience of a saint, the calmness of a monk, and an essence of an angel.

"You know I will never turn down a surprise visit," I reply, "and yes, I am ready for breakfast whenever you are, of course." Keiki used to insist I eat up here alone because she seems to think it's unprofessional to enjoy a meal with me since I pay her to be here, but the idealism behind such a thought is ridiculous. We should eat together like family. She takes care of me and helps in every way possible. The least I can do is enjoy meals with her after she spends the time preparing the food.

"Wonderful," she says, blowing me a kiss. "I'll be right back with breakfast. In the meantime, is it okay if I allow Daniel in to visit?" Keiki glances over her shoulder into the hallway. I suspect whoever Daniel is must be nearby.

Daniel? I don't think I'm acquainted with anyone by that name. He might be one of the nice sailors from down the street. They stop by from time to time to say hello. Although, he didn't resemble a sailor by the look of those fancy clothes. Gosh, sometimes my mind acts like an old record player hitting a pesky scratch. I've become so awful with names. "Of course. Send Daniel out here."

My eyes aren't bad for a woman my age, but unless I'm familiar with the sight, it's hard to make out particular details. Daniel possesses familiar features, but I can't place my finger on where I would know him from.

I adjust my position within the chair, waiting for Daniel to make his way outside. With a moment to jog through my thoughts, I can only wish there was a way to reconnect the loose wires that make up my memory.

At a closer glance, I notice Daniel is a young man and looks to be in his mid-twenties. He sure is handsome in those navy-blue pleated pressed slacks and white button-down dress shirt. There isn't one dark strand of hair out of place or a flaw within his smooth complexion. His smile encompasses a sense of weakness, or discomfort, but he appears happy to be here. I can read a person best by the appearance in their eyes though, and I see a brilliant reflection from the sun, highlighting an aura of warmth. It's easy to tell he's a pleasant fellow. Life has clearly graced me with so many wonderful people, so I'm not at all surprised.

Daniel leans over and places a kiss on my cheek. "Good morning, Gran, how are you feeling today?"

Gran? Daniel. He doesn't resemble my granddaughter, Makena, and she's the only one entitled to call me Gran. My hands tighten around my notebook as I strain to understand why this man is referring to me as his grandmother. The emptiness in my mind pains my heart. Surely, the answer must be in my head —somewhere.

What's worse is it seems I'm making Daniel uncomfortable as he appears to be searching for the guest chair. He spots the wrought-iron seat in the corner and carries it closer to me. After a moment of scratching at his cheek and adjusting his collar, he sits down and folds his hands, cupping them over his knees while leaning into his elbows.

"I'm Makena's husband." A nervous smile plays along the dimples of his cheeks. *Makena got married? She's such a young girl still.* "She's busy teaching all those classes at the university. Otherwise, she'd be here with me now, but she'll be by later, of course."

A professor. My Makena is a professor, yet no one thought to tell me.

"What does she teach, may I ask?"

Daniel fiddles with his wedding band, proof of marriage. I'm sure the memory will come back to me.

"Political Science," he says before clearing his throat.

I can't help the chuckle piping through my lungs. *A girl who takes after my heart—my granddaughter is a professor of Political Science.* The DNA in this family must run strong. "How admirable," I say, releasing a quiet sigh. "Well, what can I do for you, Daniel?" I have a habit of repeating names when I speak, so it sticks to the front of my mind while we're together.

"Hmm," he says, shifting in his seat. "I suppose my answer isn't quite that simple, but I'm hoping you might be interested in helping with an idea I have. I'm a journalist for the Tribune—the newspaper."

His pause after telling me what he does for a living leaves me wondering if he's waiting for a response. "That is lovely," I say.

Daniel smiles, but the curves along the sides of his lips flatten after a swift second. "Yes, but I'm here to ask you for your help with a piece I'm writing."

It's difficult to remember something as simple as my last name these days, so I'm not sure how I can benefit this young man, but at the very least, I will try my best. He's too polite to turn away. "What would you need from me, Daniel?"

He stretches his fingers out and grips his hands around his

notepad then exhales a lungful of air. "This coming December marks the seventy-fifth anniversary of the attack on Pearl Harbor."

Oh, my sweet Pearl.

As if an automatic response, I utter: "'A date which will live in infamy,' Roosevelt declared. He was right, wasn't he?" My heart quivers in reminiscence of hearing those words delivered through the radio. Of course, I didn't need to hear the announcement to comprehend the atrocity our country was experiencing.

"He was most certainly correct," Daniel agrees.

My short-term memory is for the birds, but my long-term memories—or most of them, are still crystal clear. "Seventy-five years," I repeat. It seems incomprehensible that so much time has passed in a blink of an eye.

Daniel drops his shoulders a touch and straightens his posture as if something I said is riveting. "I know you have some trouble with your memory, but I was wondering if you might recall a story to share with the Tribune readers?"

I would love nothing more than to tell Daniel my mind is overflowing with vivid recollections and I'm just slow at piecing them together, but I still don't recognize the poor man and I'm staring at him with such intensity, trying my best to unscramble my thoughts.

"Breakfast is here," Keiki announces as she carries a tray of fruit and pastries out onto the terrace. "Is Daniel going to be accompanying us this morning?"

The hollow feeling in my head is like a numbness—one that terrifies me some days. "Yes, please, Daniel, stay and join us for breakfast." As the words spill from my mouth, a cloud stirs through the sky, pulling my attention toward the ocean's horizon. "Are we expecting showers today?" I ask.

"Not that I'm aware," Keiki responds.

"The clouds appear different, don't they?" Odd clouds have never been a good prediction of upcoming events.

From the corner of my eye, I spot the exchange of a concerning expression between Keiki and Daniel. I recognize their silent analysis. It's one that suggests *this poor elderly woman is losing a battle with the enemy that's stealing her mind.* Young people

assume the worst about the older generation. I'm not bothered by
their presumptions since I can tell them with certainty that there
is no reason to worry about me. But it's impossible to explain a
lifetime's worth of rationale to those who haven't lived through
what I have.

2

JULY 1941

THERE'S something to say about being awake before the alarms rattle through the house. The silence embraces me with comfort and a moment to sneak in a cup of coffee before the hustle and bustle of the day begins. While watching the dribbles and droplets of deep brown liquid seep from the filter into the glass flask, my mouth waters, but staring at the hypnotic sight won't speed up the process.

The scent of French coffee grinds follows me to the front door as I release the bolted locks to welcome in the humid air, rich with blends of dew-covered blossoms. No one is outside just yet. It's still early, but the newspaper is where it is every morning, neatly rolled into a tight tube and bound with a rubber band. At least I know the paperboy is awake before I am. I pinch one end of the rolled print, avoiding the horrible ink stains I attract most days, and hold it out in front of me like a dirty sock as I close myself back into the house.

I place the paper down on the kitchen table at Dad's spot, careful not to brush it against the canary yellow place-setting. The struggle of scrubbing ink stains out of fabric never makes for a good start to the day.

My father and older twin brothers, James, and Lewis, enjoy their pancakes, bacon, and eggs more than the nectar birds outside like to sing, so I try to have everything ready before they wake up during the work week.

My hands know the routine better than my mind most days and making breakfast and setting the table occurs somewhat seamlessly, bringing me to five a.m. when the alarm clocks will wake them up.

The flask of coffee is full, and I steal the first cup before placing it on a hot mat in the center of the kitchen table.

"James, Lewis, get up, men," Dad shouts down the hallway. Lewis is most likely already up and dressed, but James has always been the slower of my brothers. He enjoys his sleep and will seize every free second before prompted out of bed—even at twenty-two years old, which is absurd.

"Morning, kiddo. Thanks for cooking up this swell breakfast." Lewis is the hungriest of us all and always the first to take a seat at the table. "Do you have any wild plans today?"

I sometimes answer this question three separate times in the morning because there isn't much else to talk about when we do the same thing every single day. "Who knows where this day will take me after class." I'm sure the tell-all smirk along my lips does little to hide the truth from Lewis, who often proves to know me better than anyone else in this house.

Despite Dad's unreasonable requests for me to stay out of certain areas on and off base, it doesn't always stop me from doing as I please. I've become tired of reminding Dad I'm a grown woman and that I selflessly stick around to help these three guys make it through a day. Mom used to be the one to keep everyone corralled, but since she's gone, I feel it's my responsibility to fill in for her.

"You're not running off to the beach today, are you?" Lewis asks in a low hush.

I glance down the hallway to see if Dad is within earshot, but the pipes are whining so he must be in the shower. "Last time I went to the beach, a lieutenant came to escort me back to base. It was humiliating. Surely, you haven't forgotten. It's hard to understand what Dad's issue is with the radius of my freedom, but something needs to change. I need to live my life." A sigh expels from my lungs, highlighting my constant frustration of living in this house. "After all, there isn't much stopping me from leaving the island once I finish my nursing classes."

Lewis quirks his lips into a smile as he stabs his fork into the stack of pancakes. "We both know you're going to stick around to watch over Dad, and besides, you must realize his only reason for the strict rules is to keep you safe. The world isn't a friendly place right now, and you are his only daughter."

"Morning," James mutters, scuffing his feet against the rusty-brown linoleum tiles. With the palms of his hands pressed against his eyelids, he groans to make a point about his distaste for being awake so early. I don't recall a day when this family has slept in, but it's clear James needs more sleep than the rest of us.

"Good morning, sunshine," I reply. "Coffee, orange juice, pancakes, bacon, and eggs?" I sound like a radio advertisement for a diner.

"Thanks, Elizabeth," James says with a curt partial smile.

I dish a serving of eggs onto his plate and stab a fork into the pile of sizzling pork. "I'll give you some extra bacon. Maybe that will perk you up," I say.

"No, no bacon."

No bacon. Okay. "Goodness, well, what about pancakes?" I continue.

"Yes, please."

I don't need to ask if he would like coffee. The answer is always a firm "yes."

"Here you go." I place his plate and mug down.

"Thanks."

With a long glance at my moody brother, I ponder why he seems grumpier than usual today. He looks disheveled. I reach over and yank at a strand of his dark, wavy hair, finding it curl over the top of his ear. "You need a haircut."

"Uh-huh." I can't tell if James needs my reminders, or if it is his intention to wait until the day before he would get into trouble with his officer, but I try to spare him the reprimand like Mom used to do.

I place Dad's dish down onto the table just as he makes his way down the hall. He likes to shower, shave, and dress before eating. Sometimes he's still chewing his food on the way out the door.

"Elizabeth, gentlemen, good morning," he addresses us. The sternness on Dad's face is a permanent fixture. His eyes appear alert, even if he's tired. His jaw is rigid—the look of a person who shows no sign of humor, and his dark hair is slick with grease to ensure no strand is out of place. Most people might see an unloving man by the looks of his cold facade, but I know better. I've become proficient at unmasking his feelings through other cues. His chest rises and falls when he's struggling internally, and his anger becomes clear during long held breaths. When he's distressed, his exhales are slow and deliberate. And though it doesn't happen often, when he's nervous, he huffs and puffs as if running a race. The only part of him I cannot decipher is when he's at peace because I don't believe he has felt that way since Mom was here.

"Good morning, Dad," I'm the first to respond.

"Morning, Sir," the twins echo one another.

For only a few brief moments, the four of us consume the food I made before the first fork pings against a glass plate. The scratching squeal from the wooden chair against the floor is next, and the dish clambering against the sink basin is the last in the sequence that will repeat twice more over the next five minutes.

"Elizabeth, your necklace," Dad says, walking away from the sink. The sound from his shoes clicks and clacks against each tile as he walks across the house toward his small work area. He retrieves a stack of paperwork and returns while skimming the front page.

I pinch my fingers around the golden Star of David, wishing Dad would stop asking me to hide who I am: a Jewish woman living in the United States during a time when other countries are at war. I don't see why I should act as if the war is in our backyard. The United States is not involved. Jewish people are not in grave danger here, and I shouldn't have to feel fear for who I am.

"Dad, people don't care what religion I practice, especially, not here on base. Don't you have enough to worry about? Please stop making such a deal out of my necklace." I can already assume his response since we have the same argument at least once a week.

"You're right, Elizabeth. No one has a problem with anyone until they do, and when they do, it's impossible to hide the truth. Why must we go over this repeatedly?" He knows why.

"It's because you know it's wrong to hide our faith. We should be proud, Jewish Americans, but we have to live in fear of a dictator who has no power over us here."

"What on earth is the matter with you? What would your mother think of this?"

"I'm sure she would tell me to wear my necklace with pride and not give more strength to those who don't deserve it."

"Elizabeth, this situation is far worse than what your mother stood her ground for. She would want you to be safe."

I couldn't be any more sheltered here, living within a gated community full of sailors, soldiers, airmen, and Marines. In fact, I'm tired of the safety. I much prefer a life outside of these walls.

With reluctance, I tuck my necklace beneath the collar of my blouse, wishing I could change how the world is controlling what I do.

"Don't forget your lunch, Dad." Egg salad, an apple, and carrot sticks are what he has been consuming for lunch every single day for as long as I can remember. I made sure not to skip a beat when Mom left us.

"Thank you, dear," Dad says, meeting me back in the kitchen. "Oh, Elizabeth, you will come straight home after class, correct?" I can give him a good line and say, yes, of course, or I can tell him the truth, which is that I have every intention of sneaking off to the beach with Audrey for a bit. "Please stay on this part of the base today, Elizabeth. I don't have the bodies to monitor you, and it's safest here."

"Yes, Sir." I allow him to treat me like a child because I don't have it in me to keep reminding him, I'm old enough to leave home, not when Mom's untimely death is still fresh, as if it just happened yesterday. He still needs me. "I'm sure I'll just spend time with Audrey, either at her house or here." He rarely has an issue with that since my closest friend lives just two houses down.

Dad leans down and places a kiss on the top of my head and

nods in James and Lewis's direction. "Men, I'm sure I'll see you later. Take care. James, haircut."

"I got it. Haircut. I know."

"Don't use that tone with me, son."

It's best if we're all quiet until we go our separate ways. Otherwise, we will have to sit through another Salzberg family feud. No one ever fought when Mom was here. I don't know how she kept everyone in line and happy, but it appeared effortless. Some days, I debate if I'll ever be able to live up to her level of perfection in maintaining a household.

3

JULY 1941

AUDREY IS WAITING at the edge of her driveway on her robin's-egg-blue bicycle. With her neatly wound victory rolls pinned above her loose auburn curls, the sheen from her styled hair offers a blinding reflection from the sun. Audrey cups her hand over her eyes as I make my way toward her, shaking her head at me with a cherry-red lined demure grin.

"How do you look so alert and perky at this hour?" Audrey asks. "Your cheeks even look pinched. I must look like a corpse in comparison."

"What a lovely thing to say, but of course, you are stunning as always," I compliment my friend.

"I think the bags beneath my eyes are growing their own bags, Lizzie. My glasses are doing nothing to hide the truth. I'll never snag a guy looking this way."

"Have you tried coffee?" I ask, knowing the drink has a power to send electrical currents through my blood.

"Oh, Lizzie, you know I can't get myself to swallow a mouthful of that disgusting beverage. It tastes like dirt."

"It could help," I offer, despite her distaste.

"The only thing that will help is to finish these darn classes."

I debate if working long shifts as a nurse rather than training in the shadows of nurses will be harder or easier. The pressure is a lot and there are always eyes on us, making sure we are conducting every move per the book. I suspect the pressure might be more when there aren't watchful gazes, though. It sure will be swell to earn a nice nickel for our work.

"Well, just a few more months. We're close." Audrey lifts her foot to the pedal, ready to get moving. "Say, what are you doing after class today?" I arch a brow to explain the reason for my question.

"Oh, dear ... no, Lizzie. Don't even say the words. You are such a troublemaker, you know that?"

"You can consider me a menace only if we get into trouble. Plus, we're grown women now. We don't need to abide by these silly rules anymore."

"My parents pay for the roof over my head. I have to follow rules," she argues.

Audrey has a point, I suppose. Until I finish these classes, moving out isn't an option. "I promise we won't get caught."

My dearest friend rolls her eyes and straightens her thick, black-framed glasses over her nose. "I'll think about it."

She's already thought about it. We both know she'll be tagging along with me after class. Neither of us can pass up the beach on a perfect day like today.

"Lizzie, why is your hair still down?" Audrey asks, stepping into her bicycle's pedals.

"Oh, Audrey, you know how I love to feel the wind blow through my locks. I have my pins. It will only take but a second to fix when we arrive."

"You sure are a pistol, Lizzie. I'll give you that."

Audrey follows the rule books down to the fine print unless my pleas become irresistible. It's not that I'm trying to set a poor example for the girl, but I feel it's far too important to deny ourselves the chance to experience our best life before we settle down, become someone's wife, and have a family. A girl simply must have fun at some point.

* * *

Our ride is brief, down the side streets along the center of Hingham Naval base. The scent of gunpowder warns us what to expect during today's field training. Murky smoke in the distance and shouts of leaders define a typical Monday morning. They must rally the boys back to their responsibilities after looking for trouble the last two days.

We take a few shortcuts to the hospital, avoiding crowds of pedestrians marching to their next destination. There is never a quiet moment to appreciate here. Life revolves around this base morning, noon, and night.

We situate our bicycles along the metal rails out in front of the emergency room entrance. Audrey secures her mode of transportation with a heavy chain and lock. I'm more of a risk taker, I suppose. I have trouble imagining anyone would take this red clunker. If they were to, it would be easier to catch them than a cow with a bell.

While Audrey snaps her lock in place, I pull the pins out of my pockets, twist the front quarters of my hair, and maneuver the strands just right to keep my face clear. "See, nothing to it, Audrey."

The motherly side-long glance I receive isn't new from my best friend. Her proof of disapproval is never far from the last time she disagreed with me.

I smear my finger beneath my lips, ensuring the red tint didn't smudge among the beads of sweat I released on our travels. "Do you want my compact?" Audrey offers.

"No, thank you. I'm sure I look fine."

Audrey and I adjust our cross-body satchels and make our way toward the main entrance of the hospital, passing no less than a dozen sailors slinging jokes and stories from their weekend.

"Good morning, ladies." One gentleman is courteous enough to pull his cigarette out from between his lips and greet us as if we're royalty crossing their path. Then, as if practiced in unison, the other boys remove their caps and tip their heads in our direction.

"Sailors," I respond with cordiality. Some of these poor fellas are just so lonely, it's no wonder the sight of a girl can cause a ripple in any conversation. However, most men should know that a female on base means they are the daughter of a higher rank, or a wife of a fellow serviceman. Still, they never falter to show their respect.

"Say, you're Commander Salzberg's daughter, aren't you now?" The question comes from behind us, and it is a common question I hear at least once a day. It is also a question I choose to ignore once a day.

"Don't ask her that, you twit," another says. The sound of a slap against skin on what I can assume to be a man's neck smarts my ears as we walk in through the glass doors of the hospital.

Rubbing alcohol and ammonia sting my nostrils as the pitter-patter of our shoes pulsate in the hallway. We're heading to the training room where Audrey, myself, and fifteen others have spent many hours over the last two-and-half years. We're considered medical volunteers until we finish our classes, but it doesn't stop the registered nurses from moving us to the front lines of this hospital when necessary. They are often short staffed and with the growing population of families on base, there is never a slow time in the wards. Our training has become real world experience, which will prepare us for the Red Cross once we finish up in a few months.

"Thank heavens," a shout rings out between the ceramic walls. "We need your help. There is a terrible virus hitting the grade school and we have a dozen children with high fevers, vomiting, and—well, you can imagine the rest, ladies. Chop, chop."

Audrey and I share a fleeting look before we hustle down the hallway toward the clean room to scrub up and mask our faces. "Poor little ones," I say, securing my apron.

"If there are twelve today, it's safe to assume there will be twice as many by tomorrow morning, Lizzie. This is terrible."

I want to help people get well, tend to the slick, mend the injured, but watching a person spew their guts—it is my weakness, one I must hide as it literally makes me green in the face.

"This is going to be a doozy," I reply.

Holy Mackerel. The children's ward doesn't have an empty bed in sight. There must be an entire classroom full of kids in here.

"There's a stomach virus going around. Many of the youngsters have high-level fevers. We need to keep cool compresses on their heads. There are buckets by each bed for bodily fluids, but you will oversee the process of switching out the dirty bins for clean ones," Nurse Jones says to us, breathless with an obvious sense of anxiousness.

It's unusual to find myself in a situation when I'm not eager to jump in and begin helping in every way possible, but there are only two nurses in the room and they seem to be in a tizzy, spinning in circles. The children are suffering, and most are very pale and shivering.

"Audrey, you can start on that side and I'll begin over here," I say.

Audrey jolts across the room and tends to the first bed while I do the same. The first young boy has sun-bleached hair, but the color of his skin is even fairer than his hair. He doesn't seem in distress like some others. Instead, he's staring out the tall window behind us. I take a moment to look at his paperwork, finding his name and age.

"Philip, my name is Elizabeth. How are you feeling?" Philip doesn't respond right away. He pins his gaze to the window. According to his paperwork, his fever is mild, but he was complaining of belly pain earlier and seems lethargic. "Are you nine years old?" I wait a moment for any sign that he might answer, but he doesn't budge. "Does your tummy hurt?"

I comb my fingers through Phillip's hair to gain his attention, which works well. Like an electrifying shock, Philip bolts up straight and clutches his arms around his abdomen. I lunge for the bucket beside his bed, catching a stomach full of bile just in the nick of time. I close my eyes throughout the duration of the heaving to avoid the sight. It's easier said than done, to breathe in and out through my mouth, as advised by the nurses teaching our classes, but I grit my teeth and wait for Philip to lay back down into his pillow.

"I think I'm better now," he says, his voice scratchy and guttural.

"Here, sweetie, let me pour you a glass of water." I spin around, finding a pitcher of water next to a row of glasses. The unsettling sensation in my gut is passing, but I must still dispose of the waste. I wish I could shut off all my senses because I can't let the nurses see my weakness. I'll never pass these classes if I'm unable to handle a little vomit.

The smells and sounds wane for a few hours, but it takes one slip of a bucket and an uncontrolled reflex to find my uniform covered.

My stomach has never been strong. I think some people are born with weak gag reflexes and the lack of ability to put mind over matter. I feel it coming. *The sympathy nausea.* First, it's the tight feeling in my throat. Then my gut spins like a merry-go-round. The ten-seconds I might have between this moment and the cause of an additional unsterile situation isn't long enough. A clean bucket is in view and I run outside of the ward and into the hallway before mimicking the sickness I have been watching all morning.

I feel better almost instantly, but I'm unsure of the scene I caused, or the protocol for when a nurse falls ill on duty. It's something I hope to learn about before finishing these classes, but for now, my only thought is to find my way to the lavatory.

"Elizabeth?" Audrey's voice echoes down the hall. "Are you all right, dear?" I pivot on the heels of my shoes while continuing to walk away and shake my head. Audrey takes one quick gander at my uniform and lifts her hand to her mouth. Her eyes widen when she notices the way I look. "Oh, my."

It's hard to move fast when trying to avoid contact with the bodily fluids covering my attire, but when Audrey finds me in the ladies' room with a toothbrush and clean clothes curled under her arm, the urge to hug her almost outweighs the recollection of what I look like. She takes a step back before I get too close. "I can't thank you enough, Audrey. I'm not sure I want to imagine what the nurses must think of me right now."

Audrey places her hand on my back as I lean over the sink and cup handfuls of water up to my mouth. "It happens to everyone. We're all human, Lizzie."

"People view nurses as heroes and women who hold a reputation for being capable of handling anything that comes their way," I say while staring at my mirroring reflection. "Audrey, I don't know if I'm cut out for this line of work." Audrey's eyes meet mine as we stare quietly at the mirror. Her eyebrows knit together, showing me a hint of sympathy, an expression she wouldn't want to put into words.

"This is the reason we are going through training, right? You mustn't let one incident bring you down, sweetie."

It's only happened once, but it could occur again. I'm not confident I will have control over my stomach any better the next time. I'm a failure and haven't become a registered nurse yet.

"We best get back to the ward. I have no business tending to myself when all of those children are so sick." I imagine being in here will only make matters worse in the eyes of the nurses.

"Well now, no need to worry. They called two nurses in to assist, and nurse Jones pardoned us for the rest of today's training. She suggests I make sure you arrive home in one piece."

"That's just marvelous," I snap, dropping my hands to the white porcelain.

"Oh, good gracious, Elizabeth. Come on, we'll stop at the store so I can make you some soup, and it will be like none of this happened."

"You don't have to do this, Audrey. I can make it home on my own, but I appreciate the offer." It's a hard pill to swallow, thinking I'm unfit to be a nurse before my career even begins. If Nurse Jones assumes I can't find my way two miles down the road, I'm sure every other staff member of this hospital must see me in the same light.

4

CURRENT DAY - OCTOBER 2018

Lost in my thoughts while staring at the deep blue sky, I turn my face away from the blinding sun, finding a man sitting beside me. My hand flies up to my chest, startled by his presence.

"Oh my, I'm so sorry. I didn't realize I had company and here I am gazing at the ocean like a seagull looking for a snack," I say, my cheeks filling with warmth from embarrassment.

"It's unnecessary to apologize. We should all take a minute to drink in this gorgeous scenery now and then. In fact, Makena seems to have most of her daydreams while sitting on the beach. It must be genetic," the fellow says with a gentle smile.

"Oh, you know my granddaughter?" I ask the handsome gentleman. I don't recall when this fellow arrived or who he is, but he seems very curious.

The man looks perplexed by my question, but I assume he understands what I'm asking since he mentioned Makena's name.

"It's me, Daniel," he says. "I'm Makena's husband."

Husband. I spot my journal on the table in front of me and open it to the last page to find the notes I must have left for myself, but it's difficult to make heads or tails of my chicken scratch. When did my penmanship become so sloppy?

"Oh yes, of course," I say in response.

"I've been interviewing you for an article about Pearl Harbor's seventy-fifth anniversary. If it's too much, we can stop or take a break," Daniel says. He's so kind and sweet, but I don't recognize him at all.

"Yes, please, continue."

Daniel takes a long moment to stare at me as if I might change my mind, but then returns his gaze to his notebook. "You must have been grateful for your education and competence in your nursing skills when the attack occurred. What would you say was the most helpful lesson you had learned prior to the chaos of that day?"

I can't seem to stop myself from staring through Daniel, as if the answer to his question is somewhere behind him. "Oh my. If I knew what I was in for when I decided on a nursing career, I might have thought twice about my decision. I couldn't handle a sick youngster; never mind the atrocities I would encounter."

"A sick child is much different from—"

Daniel's face becomes blurry as I recall a grown man crying out for his mother.

He was a grown man, per the US Navy, but he couldn't have been over eighteen—still a child. He would not make it. I was sure. The explosion engulfed his body with flames, and yet he survived the explosive that hit his ship. "I need to say goodbye to my mother, please," he cried.

"You will see your mother again," I wrongfully promised, but I couldn't bear to steal his hope when it was all he had left. His burns were too severe and covered his entire body. He was melting in front of my eyes.

"I love her so much," the boy whimpered. "She was braver than me. I'm not very brave at all, am I, nurse?"

"You are very courageous, and you are just like your mother. I promise you she is proud of the man you have grown into," I told him.

I'm not sure where the words came from, being a young girl myself without the experience of a mother, but it felt like the right thing to say as I watched the boy take his last breath.

"Not quite," I respond to Daniel. "I knew I had a lot to learn before I could become a certified practicing nurse. There was no room for weakness, and that day was far from an exception."

Daniel presses his pen down to his notepad and glances up at me. "Everyone is weak or faint of heart at some point. That's what makes us all human, but time, knowledge and wisdom help us work around our inadequacies, I suppose."

"To fall helpless at the sight of a sick child was not a moment I could sweep under the carpet, not then."

"Well, how did you go about overcoming your weakness?" he asks.

"Watching a man take his last breath changes the way the world appears. The knowledge and feeling of being powerless enforces perseverance because there's no other choice."

5

JULY 1941

WE APPROACH the front doors of the commissary, but Audrey hesitates. "I'm not sure I want to know what I look like at the moment," she says, smoothing her hands down the sides of her hair. To be imperfect when walking into a store is what some ladies find to be a sin, but the both of us were in the trenches of an atrocious viral outbreak this morning.

To Audrey's credit, her hair has slipped from its pins, and the moisture in the air has added an abundance of volume to her barrel waves but upon a closer look, I notice her creamy beige eyeshadow and mascara are a bit smudged, and the lipstick she reapplied several times today has faded to her natural pink pigment. I can only imagine the way I must appear. At least Audrey has dark hair and complementing lashes and eyebrows. The coloring of my features matches the strawberry blonde hue of my hair. I imagine I look sicker than I did an hour ago.

"Let's cross our fingers we don't run into anyone we know," Audrey says, peeping around the outside of the store as if we're doing something that could land us in hot water.

"Two paper bags might come in handy," I tease.

Audrey places her finger beneath her chin, appearing to be thinking about my suggestion. "Well, it isn't the worst idea," she replies. "At least we still have time before the afternoon rush."

The commissary is busiest at three unconventional times

during the day. For the first two hours, the place fills up with ambitious women, who have a solid plan for the day.

Then, just after lunch, women with children in school try to finish the last of their errands before the kids come home.

The third group arrives just after completing their daily duties. These are the unmarried men who conduct their weekly shopping in increments without a pre-planned list.

Dad detests when I end up at the commissary around the last busy hour of the day. Of course, he's aware of the unwritten fairy tales that take place at a grocery store—it's said to be where every fairytale love story begins. I know Dad wants nothing more than for me to find a suitable husband to settle down with, but per his absurd request, the man of my unknown dreams shall not live on this military base.

His explanations have never been clear, why he opposes the idea of me falling in love with one of the qualified young men he works beside daily, but I haven't argued the point with him since I am in no rush to settle down. Dad doesn't understand my independent side yet. He feels that a girl my age should fret about their biological clock, but he doesn't want me to feel that way about a man who might face a deployment at any unsuspecting minute. In any case, I'm not in the same hurry as the others. I don't believe the world will run out of husbands any time in the future.

Audrey, however, doesn't feel the same. She is sure there is a shortage of men, or at least decent ones, and she's worried all the other women will sweep them up first. Audrey has been on the prowl for quite some time. I watch her wandering eye whenever we're out, inspecting every potential bachelor with a romantic fantasy swirling around in her mind. More times than not, she finds something wrong with each eligible man she spends over five minutes with. If I've told her once, I've told her a thousand times to quit being so fussy, let loose, and have a little fun since we're only twenty once in life, but my words go in one ear and out the other.

As we were hoping, the commissary is somewhat empty. The store clerks have realigned all the buggies and hand-held baskets to prepare for the next rush of customers. Audrey and I each take a basket and loop the metal handle around our arms.

"I can take care of your items. You shouldn't be carrying so much weight around after upchucking your breakfast, Lizzie."

It would be awkward to gallivant around the store without a buggy or a basket. No one comes in here to browse, and I don't know if I've met a woman who has left this store with less than a handful of items. "You're overreacting, Audrey. As you can see, I'm fine now."

Audrey sets her gloved palm on my cheek. "Dear, you are still white as a ghost. I insist you allow me to help. You know, it's all right to take a hand when offered sometimes."

"Well, I know better than to argue with you, so I appreciate your kindness. Thank you. I won't put much in my basket," I assure her.

While strolling through the aisles, the memory of why we came here in the first place nearly slips my mind. Though by the sight of Audrey's basket, she hasn't forgotten a thing. Soup. That's right. She has more than enough ingredients to boil a pot of soup.

"Oh, just one more thing that will fix you up. You can't have soup without crackers when you're sick. Then we'll be ready to check out," Audrey says, holding up a finger and pivoting on her heels. I drag my tired legs behind her but stop when I hear a hushed conversation from the next aisle over.

"Shirley, did you notice who is here?" a woman asks.

I peer over to Audrey, curious if she caught wind of the nearby chatter. The crease between her eyebrows confirms she heard the same whisper, so we lean our ears in toward the stacked shelves, hoping to catch more of what might be juicy gossip.

"Who on earth are you talking about, Greta?" The discussion becomes harder to hear but continues from just a few feet and a wall of coffee grounds away. If only I could get another foot closer, I could find out what they're saying. But if I lean in any further, I may become one with the shelves of tin canisters.

"Evidently, Everett Anderson is relocating to this base."

Everett Anderson. The mention of this name is so startling that I lose my balance. No matter what I try to reach for, it falls with me. Even though Audrey lunges for my arm as a last attempt to prevent what's about to happen, I only end up pulling her down too.

A round of crashes, clangs, and shrieks blare through the store as the shelves moan and croak, tilting into the next aisle. I thank the heavens above when the display shelves catch on the surrounding ones, keeping the racks from falling to the ground. Only the shelf-lined products fell, but they landed right on top of the poor ladies who were having a private chat.

Once I'm able to right myself, I rush to the next aisle with my hands cupped over my mouth. "I am so deeply sorry for falling into the shelves. Ladies, is everyone all right?"

I reach over to the shoulder of the woman closest to me. Her right palm is on her chest and the other hand is against the shelf that was about to crash down. The second woman is already frantic about working to tidy up the mess of cereal boxes.

"Goodness, gracious. I am terribly sorry. You see, I had become ill earlier and my dear friend Audrey was trying to collect items to make me a pot of soup. I must have fallen dizzy again. How embarrassing," I continue gabbing, hoping one of the two will say something, anything at all.

"You scared me silly." The woman isn't much older than me, but by the wedding band outline beneath her brown fitted gloves, I assume she's a housewife shopping during an off hour. "Gerta," she says, introducing herself as she removes her hand from her chest.

"Gerta, again, I apologize for frightening you. I'm Elizabeth."

"Oh sure, now I know why you look familiar. I've seen you around," the other woman, who I suspect to be Shirley, states. "You are Commander Salzberg's daughter, yes?"

My instinct is to shush her, so no one else in this store hears our conversation. Though, it would serve me right after eavesdropping.

"Yes, I am—his daughter," I reply as if insulted by the question.

"I'm Shirley. It's a pleasure to meet you, Elizabeth," she says.

Audrey scurries around the corner, eyeballing me as if she lost a small child two aisles away. "There you are. I thought you might have gotten sick again." At least her words place extra merit on my tall tale. "You see ..." Audrey chuckles while catching her breath, "Elizabeth, here, got wind—"

My interruption is abrupt, keeping Audrey from completing her sentence.

"Of a fleeting smell that knocked me off my feet," I say. "Thank goodness Audrey caught me before I went down."

"A smell?" Shirley repeats. "What in the world could smell so awful?"

"I—uh, there was an open can of sardines—"

Audrey gives me a hard side-glance with yet another motherly glare.

"Anyway," I snicker, while corralling as many items into my arms as I can hold. "I'll take care of this. You ladies have a lovely afternoon now."

"Oh dear, don't be a fool. We're all okay, and if there's one thing we're efficient at, it's cleaning up messes," Greta says with what sounds like forced laughter.

Does anyone want to be *good* at cleaning? It doesn't seem like much of an accomplishment, but this is the stuff women say to one another as a testament to their achievement of being an outstanding homemaker. Being proficient in tidying up disarray makes me extra sure that marriage is not something I want to rush into.

"Ladies, ladies, is everyone good here? I was searching every aisle for where the racket came from."

The four of us stand here doe-eyed, with rather senseless gazes toward the man standing just a couple of feet away. My mouth falls ajar, and I'm not sure if I can remember how to use my manners now.

The long-winded sigh expelling from my lungs doesn't help the situation, but—his smile, it's as white as it appeared on film and in the magazines. Everett's alluring hooded eyes glisten, but I didn't know they were a minty-green until now, and his hair is the color of coffee and milk, which differs from the inky black strands I assumed he had. The coloring in the magazines makes everything look a little different. This man is even taller and broader than he appeared—far more handsome than Hollywood depicts.

"Ladies?" he questions, sounding unsure of himself this time. I realize a full minute must have passed since he already asked us if we were okay. It's obvious we are all star-struck, standing before this familiar man in his unfamiliar army pinks and greens uniform. He must have joined the Army Air Corps. The branch is brand new, and the uniforms are different—quite striking, in fact.

"Yes, yes, we are just fine. Thank you so much for checking on us ... Lieutenant," I respond after inspecting the rank patches on his sleeve. "I've been a big, old klutz today, and I knocked a few items off the shelf. One minute I'm minding my business and then there was a—a smell, and suddenly, everything came crashing down. I sure know how to make a big uproar." I shouldn't have been the one to answer his question, since I'm likely the only one of the four who has a nasty habit of talking in circles, but it's too late.

"You knocked over the entire row of shelves," Audrey mutters between her pressed lips.

Everett inspects Audrey then the other two women before returning his jewel-like eyes to my big mouth.

"The entire row?" he counters.

"Well, not, as you can see." I wave my hand at the cereal boxes as if my arm is a magic wand.

"We—we th—thought it was a rumor that you were living on the base now," Greta says, stuttering through her words.

I cannot convince myself that Everett Anderson, a Hollywood heartthrob, is standing here in the commissary on this tiny island. The odds are almost unreal.

"A rumor?" He chuckles at the statement. "No, more like a secret. I was quiet about my move and the decision to switch careers over the last year. I don't believe everything needs to be public knowledge."

"You left Hollywood to join the Army?"

"The Army Air Corps," I correct Shirley.

"Yes, Ma'am. Hollywood doesn't fulfill a man's desire to protect and defend his country." I'm not sure how someone who must have everything could still feel a lack of accomplishment. "Ladies, if I may—could I ask a small favor of you?"

The four of us say, "Yes," in melodic harmony.

"Do you think you could keep my whereabouts a secret? The other fellas don't seem to know who I am. At least it seems most of them don't. I'm enjoying the freedom from fame." A wry smirk grows along his perfect lips, as if he's shy about his reputation. His cheeks even blush a little. He sure is something. A dreamboat, as I've called him in the past.

"Of course," we agree, repeating each other once again as we all nod our heads at the same second.

It's only a matter of time before he's spotted by someone who recognizes him, but with as kind as he was to search for whatever trouble he thought was going on here, the least we can do is keep quiet about our encounter. "It was nice to meet you all."

I know my imagination plays tricks on me now and again, but his last glance before roaming away was most definitely toward me.

The moment Everett Anderson is out of sight, the four of us fan ourselves as if we have been slaving over a stove for hours.

"How are we supposed to keep this a secret?" Gerta asks. I'm not surprised she's the first one to ask since she was the one who started the initial whisper of gossip to begin with.

"I'm sure it's the least we can do for a gentleman giving up his freedom for our country," I say. Acting superior to other women on base isn't a wonderful quality, but I should protect this innocent man and adhere to his plea of silence.

"Right, absolutely," Gerta agrees with a hint of snideness along her pinched smirk. "I'm glad you are all right, and I'm all right. All of us are fine and dandy, so I suppose we should get back to our womanly obligations now. Have a good day, ladies," she says, taking Shirley by the elbow while brushing past us.

When a moment of quiet and clarity returns, I realize how *under the weather* I must look after my day with a group of vomiting children, and Audrey—her hair is still a mess. I run my fingers beneath my eyes, hoping my mascara hasn't smudged too much, but my finger is far from clean when I check for damage. Audrey cups her hands around her hair and her eyes grow wide.

"Of all the days and times," she says with wide eyes, "we run into a famous picture person looking like this?"

"Well, I'm positive we left a lasting impression on him," I reply.

"We would have been better off with paper bags, Lizzie." Audrey pats her hand down the sides of her hair once more and reclaims the basket from the floor. "I still need to grab the crackers. Why don't you meet me at the checkout counter?"

With my empty basket, I allow my eyes to wander while making my way up to the front of the store. I bet he already left. He seems like a man who knows what he wants and can find it fast. Although being new to the base, I can't imagine he knows his way around the store all that well.

I peek down the aisle across from the checkout counter, finding the area empty. However, when I turn back to the space in front of me, I find a life size display of Spam. The store clerks stacked all the cans to perfection. They are set into a solid column, one on top of another until I stumble into it. I catch the two falling from the top, grateful to be spared of another mortifying situation. Of course, my gratitude must not have been loud enough as several more cans of Spam fall while I attempt to replace the first two.

"Audrey," I call out, trying to keep my voice down so I don't attract any extra attention. "Sweetie, could you give me a quick hand?" My question doesn't sound as calm as I intended.

"It seems you aren't having a splendid afternoon."

I clench my eyes and grit my teeth into a smile. Mr. Hollywood is behind me, witnessing another ruckus. He takes the cans I'm holding against the display and places them back in their proper spots before straightening another few that might fall. "Are you sure you're okay, Miss?"

"Oh yes, I'm swell. Today has been a day for the birds, that's all." And now I'm staring at this man like a hungry lion waiting for supper. I don't stare at men like they are gods of the Greek world. I don't believe in drooling over sweet talk or perfect smiles. Plus, if I did, and I met him here of all places, Dad would close the door on the subject and the guy quicker than I could accept a date.

With nerves firing through me like short circuits, I pull my hands away from the display, hoping it's safe to move without causing more damage. Then I watch Everett's gaze float across my left hand.

"Say, I'm new around here. By any chance, would you have any interest in joining me for dinner? Maybe you could share a few tips about this island?"

I suppose this is how it's done. This is how a man asks a woman out. I wouldn't know because of the relentless fear that half of this base has for Dad, but I am certain Lieutenant Anderson isn't familiar with Commander Salzberg. Not yet anyway.

I can't help but allow my distraught stare to fall to the floor between us.

"Lieutenant, it's kind of you to ask, but I don't think—"

"You are already someone's girl," he says, assuming what I was about to say.

I lift my head and stifle a soft laugh. "Oh, no, I'm nobody's girl, but I'm afraid you might not find my company to be in your best interest."

It isn't hard to understand the reason his dark shaped eyebrows are almost touching each other. "I apologize for not understanding, but I'm sure you have a good reason."

It isn't a good reason at all. I would love nothing more than to join *the* Everett Anderson for dinner, but I would have to break rules—rules I have chosen not to flirt with before.

"Well, maybe I'll see you around sometime."

"That would be lovely," I reply.

It would.

6

JULY 1941

IN THE AFTERNOONS, when I walk my bicycle down the street from Audrey's house, I sometimes imagine Mom still sitting on the front stoop waiting for me to come home from school. She would have the newspaper held open in front of her, wearing her tinted circular sunglasses and a floral print dress, looking every bit the part of a Naval lieutenant's wife on the outside.

Mom and Dad were in a loving relationship, but Mom had an aversion with the Navy's lifestyle. Despite her desire to live differently and frustration toward specific military rules, she would always tell me: "When we love someone, we will move mountains with them and for them."

I never asked if she felt like she loved Dad more than he loved her, but the thought crossed my mind from time to time. If she was unhappy living here on base, I don't understand why he never considered changing careers. She was never quiet about her opinions within the confines of our home, but never spoke out of turn when in public. In fact, I recall spotting a certain flare in her eyes when we were around others, and she would agree with statements I know she didn't want to comply with. There were times her right eyebrow would lift into the slightest arch, as if she wanted to argue a point but wouldn't dare.

Dad tells me I'm just like her whenever I dispute his beliefs on a specific subject. Mom never backed down. Her determination was a force to bear, and her strength and courage were something I could only hope I too possessed. But, when Dad compares me to her, I know he's suggesting that my powerful will and argumentative nature would be my downfall, resulting in a similar outcome like the one that befell Mom. On the contrary, some might say the same about him. Every man living on base spends their days preparing for the unthinkable, when so many countries are at war.

I gasp when entering through the front door of our house, not expecting to see Dad sitting upright on his favorite chair with a cold scowl. The sun's glare leaking in through the bay window spears his left eye, but he refuses to blink. He's angry. It's obvious.

"You're home early." The less I say, the easier these conversations are, so I turn to hang my satchel on the coat hook.

"According to the hospital staff, you should have been here over two hours ago," he says, peering down at his watch to highlight his statement.

I weave my fingers together and squeeze my knuckles through frustration. "Dad, I think we need to have a talk."

"Pardon me?" His response doesn't allow me enough time to complete my sentence.

I pull my heels off, one at a time, reveling in the desirable expansion of my toes after scrunching them into the narrow tips of my shoes all day. I'm stalling to recenter my thoughts. Nothing I say will go over well with him.

Dad cups a hand over each of his knees and waits for my response with a clear look of impatience.

"I am twenty years old, which means I'm at an age where I could consider marriage and living elsewhere. While you continue to treat me like a child, I think you should understand the facts. I choose to live here because I don't have the heart to leave the three of you, knowing you have no one to take care of the house and prepare your meals while you're at work all day."

We have gone around in circles with this conversation in the past, but I never seem to get my point across. It's a cycle of arguments without a solution. Dad tilts his head to the side and juts his chin out.

"I must have missed the part where you tell me you met a man who will take care of you and ask for your hand in marriage. Do you have the means to support yourself outside of this house?"

Our disagreements have no resolution. Until I finish school, we both know I don't have the qualifications to earn an income. Therefore, I have nowhere to go. "It doesn't have to be this way, Dad. I'm a young woman now, not the child you treat me as."

"Elizabeth, you are my daughter, and I will care for you until the day I die. If you don't understand this as a young woman, I am sure someday when you are a mother, you might feel the same, and only then agree with me on the matter."

Sometimes I wish Dad would stand up and let out all his anger, yell, or even slam a door. His complacent responses are infuriating. It feels as though he doesn't care to see life from my perspective. "I have never questioned your love for me, but you have to allow me to live and learn. I don't want to be a piece of property owned by this family until I'm passed onto a man who will call me his wife and treat me the same way. Why can't you understand this?"

Dad shifts his position, leaning from the left to right. "A piece of property? Is that what they call a daughter these days?"

"That is how I feel. Men look at women as if they deserve us—a housekeeper, a cook, a caretaker. I don't want to live this way. I want more. In fact, I want to be unforgettable."

Dad is silent for a moment. It's as if he needs to review my remarks to figure out what I'm saying, but no matter how I explain my feelings, he often perceives my words as nothing more than gibberish. "I don't know where this idealism is coming from, but I hope you are keeping these thoughts to yourself, Elizabeth. Women work hard to maintain a home for their families. Women are the ones we, as men, depend on to keep us fed and cared for when we aren't working. Without women, we would be helpless souls. To see yourself as anything less than someone who will support a man in that way is disappointing to hear."

Isn't it obvious by the efforts I put forth that I am capable of more than cooking and cleaning? His mindset is set in a time that many women want to move away from.

"You haven't had a wife in five years. You are still eating nicely prepared meals and living in a clean house. Am I wrong?"

He knows I have been filling Mom's role. My life came to a halt after her death, and to make matters worse, I often feel unappreciated. For this reason, Dad should view me as a more mature woman than most others my age, but there is no incentive for him to see me as any more than a girl who lost her mother at fifteen and took over as the matriarch to ensure the care continues for our family every day.

"I know life hasn't been easy for any of us, Elizabeth. You have done more than I could ask of you over the last five years, but regardless of how thankful I am for your strength and willingness to keep our family together, I will not stop worrying about you. You might as well ask me to stop breathing."

Dad and I stare at each other for a long moment, both of us realize how his words came out. "I didn't mean to say—"

"I understand."

Dad's focus drops to his lap, making sure I can't read the look within his eyes. Yet, I know he's disappointed in himself. "I heard you became ill at the hospital earlier. Are you feeling better now?"

"I'm fine."

"Okay then, I will handle dinner this evening. Why don't you go rest?"

As usual, we are back to where we started when I walked through this door. I'm still a woman with no authority or say over my life, and he is still a man who doesn't know his way around a kitchen which means we will eat Spam for supper if I don't intervene.

It's clear we both need a few minutes to cool down, but as I excuse myself from his pointed stare, he holds up his forefinger. "I heard you met Mr. Anderson today."

"I don't know what or who you are talking about."

"Elizabeth Salzberg, he is a troubled man. Do not underestimate the power of the rich. There is a reason he left Hollywood to join the Army Air Corps."

A fleeting moment of hostility fires through me as I wonder who has so little to do, they felt the need to inform Dad whose path I crossed at the commissary. "I wasn't aware you were familiar with Everett Anderson."

Dad stands from his chair and straightens his belt. "The captain briefed us regarding his arrival."

"What for?" I press.

"Do you have any idea what kind of attention he will attract to this area? It's the last thing this base needs. All we can hope for is that his presence here doesn't become another unneeded tourist attraction."

"You're faulting a man for changing his career path?"

Dad stares down at me from eight inches above my head. He and the twins are all six feet tall and hover over me. "No man runs away from a money pit unless he has a good reason, Elizabeth. If he thinks the military is better suited for him than Hollywood, he is in for a shock. Just, stay away, do you understand?"

It doesn't matter who I keep a distance from because there isn't a single guy on this base who would come within ten feet of me, knowing who my father is. No one is that stupid. "I'm sure it's nothing you need to worry about, Dad."

"It's nothing I should have to worry about, Elizabeth. You don't know what's going on out there right now. I can't afford any trouble from you, so I hope I am making myself clear."

I know not to ask questions about what may or may not be happening "out there" because anything Dad knows is confidential and he cannot discuss it with me. It's an understanding I've grown up with and one I won't tempt or question, but his hints and remarks make my thoughts run wild with wonder sometimes.

7

JULY 1941

WHEN I STARE into the mirrored slab stretched along the lavatory wall, I wonder how I got to this point—this stagnant moment which could look the same day after day, year after year. All that will change will be the deepening lines across my forehead and crow's feet perching out from the sides of my eyes. I won't have a choice but to cut my bangs to cover the signs of aging. I've seen what this hospital does to a nurse. She carries the weight of many lives on her shoulders, never slouching, never groaning, or wincing at an ache from standing in heels for hours each day. A nurse is a superhuman who saves lives but also smiles when squatting down to a child's level to hand out a sucker. How can one person be so many things? Mom was under the assumption she could take on the world, save everyone, leave no one behind, but then it seemed like she was the one who stayed behind. Her death wasn't the classic definition of a sacrifice, not compared to what our military men give up, but she chose others over herself and it was a sacrifice—one she made on our entire family's behalf.

I once swore to myself I wouldn't follow in her footsteps or desert my family for the greater good. In fact, I must have scribbled this statement into my diary more than a hundred times. My anger toward life was getting the best of me after Mom died, but in truth, I want nothing more than to be just like her.

When the time came for me to decide, Mom's voice found me in the darkness of night.

Alone, gazing at the sight of the moon kissing its reflection against the horizon, I wondered if I had my thoughts wrong. I contemplated whether I should become a nurse or a journalist. I didn't know if my life's focus should be on self-fulfillment or the deed of doing good for others.

It was a question no one could answer, but Mom's last words swept through my mind like a blast of cool air. It was as if she was standing before me, holding my chin within her warm, gentle hand.

"But I saved so many, Elizabeth."

The drawn-out sound of whispering syllables brought a chill to my spine. Each word was clear and crisp, harmonizing with the orchestra of crashing waves. I twisted around, searching from right to left, behind me and toward the tide, convinced I wasn't alone.

In contrast, I had never felt lonelier, but a sense of clarity overcame me.

If I was to become a journalist rather than a nurse, I may never make an impact on the world, let alone one person. My words could become lost in an attic somewhere, and that option isn't enough for what I desire in life. I want to leave my footprint here, which means my words would offer more while caring for and comforting the wounded and sick.

I pull out my tube of lipstick and brighten the red tint on my lips before returning to the training room. With a quick blot on a tissue, I smile to check for smudges and lead the click clacking echo from my heels out into the corridor.

Just before entering the training room, I spot about a dozen soldiers pushing through the main entrance of the hospital. I can only imagine what has happened.

We were in the process of a lecture on the effects of Penicillin but none of the other students are sitting in their seats, which tells me there's an all-hands-on deck issue. Two of the teaching nurses are chatting with hushed voices, and I spot Audrey conversing with a co-trainee. "It looks like there is another viral infection on the prowl. What's today's story?"

"A test flight exercise didn't go as planned. Someone mentioned the possibility of a gear failing just after takeoff."

"How many injuries in total?" I ask.

Judy, one of the other nurses in training, turns to peek at the nurses across the room. It seems she has information she's not allowed to share, but if we're supposed to help, we should know what happened. "There were two men in the aircraft. The pilot landed the plane without significant damage, but there were soldiers training nearby. Some of them took hits from flying debris and shrapnel. From what I could overhear, the men sustained only superficial injuries—nothing very serious. However, there appears to be confidential information regarding the incident, so I'm not sure about our involvement yet."

Audrey's eyes widen into the shapes of almonds. She stares at me as if I should be able to read her expression, but that only adds to the confusion.

"Ladies, we are going to be using some hands-on experience with superficial wounds today. Sutures might be necessary, but I have faith that you are prepared with steady hands. As a reminder, anything you see or hear today shall remain confidential under all circumstances. We have to protect our men's privacy at all costs."

We have been through this one crucial rule since the first day we began training, but I don't think I've attended one session where this reminder hasn't come up. It may be more difficult for those who didn't grow up on base or in a military lifestyle. I understand these rules all too well, which offers me an advantage in certain situations. It's well known the nursing staff can trust me, as well as Audrey, due to our family ties to the military.

"We will assign a pair of assisting hands to each triage bed along with necessary medical records. Do any of you have any questions for me?" Nurse Jones asks.

We have had extensive training with sutures, superficial wounds, and burns. Dealing with a room full of vomiting children will make this situation seem easy in comparison.

"No, Ma'am," I respond, following the others.

"Lizzie and Audrey, bed nine," she assigns.

The closer we walk toward triage the more laughter and boisterous sounds echo down the corridor. "They don't sound to be in rough shape," Audrey says. Her forehead wrinkles with confusion. "Is this a joke to them?"

"My dad always says: 'If you can't learn to laugh at what's thrown at you, then it will laugh at you.' It makes sense, I guess," I tell her.

Audrey twists her head and lowers her glasses down the bridge of her nose to give me a pointed look. "No, that statement doesn't make much sense at all."

"They need to lighten up a bit, is all I'm trying to say. I wish my dad would do so. Trust me."

"I can understand all too well," she says. Our dads are comrades and friends with many similar traits, or lack thereof, I should say. They're both quiet, emotionless, and stale.

We stroll down the row of triage beds and I'm having trouble spotting some injuries as we pass by, but that doesn't mean much. Bed nine is a bit of a doozy, though. A strip of gauze is sagging from the top right of the man's head, down to the left corner of his chin. His knuckles are bleeding through the gauze wrapped around both hands too. "Goodness, it looks like you might have seen the worst of this, Sir," I say, inspecting the dressing taped to his head a little closer. The gauze is overlapping his eyes, but there doesn't seem to be damage to the front of his face.

"I was the one flying the plane," he says, his voice hoarse and choky, yet vaguely familiar. "Nothing feels too serious, though."

"On you or the plane?" I offer a small smile, unsure if he can see me beneath the gauze.

"Very funny, Miss. The plane has seen better days, but I don't believe I have any broken bones. Just a laceration on the side of my face, and my hands from some shattered glass."

Audrey is preparing the supplies to clean up the wounds as I nervously prepare to remove the temporary dressing.

With a gentle tug, I strip the tape free from the man's hair, causing a mist of glass dust to fall from his hazelnut strands. He winces at the tug against his hair, and I'm worried for how much everything else might hurt. With a gradual slow movement, I peel the gauze away from his face. There is little resistance, which is a good thing. It isn't until I uncover his eyes that I see the true damage and confirm my assumptions. My mouth falls open as if I'm facing a shocking scene.

"Oh my—it's you—" I clear my throat to rectify my blundering acknowledgment. "Pardon me—aloha, Lieutenant Anderson." I salute the Hollywood star, still struck with disbelief to find him sitting before me. There is minimal damage to his face aside from an-inch-long laceration on his temple. The injury was deep and I'm not sure there isn't still glass lodged. "Are you in a lot of pain?"

He smirks and glances up at me. "Well, now, I recognize you," he says with a grin. "But, no, Miss, I feel much less sore now that you're tending to me."

He's a famous charmer. How could I forget? "Do you say that to all the nurses you run into?" Not that I'm a certified nurse yet, but for all intents and purposes, I'm acting on behalf of one.

"I don't come into contact with many nurses," he says. "Believe it or not, I try to stay out of trouble." It's inconceivable that this man with beautiful eyes and a charming smile tries to stay out of trouble. I can only imagine what type of shenanigans he attracts.

Audrey clears her throat, trying to hand me the supplies to irrigate the wound. I forgot she was standing behind me. I jump and spin around with my hands open. She shakes her head at me with disdain and I take the instruments. "Let me know if this becomes uncomfortable at any point," I say.

It's already more than uncomfortable in here for me, but I must remain composed and professional. While cleaning the lacerated area, I find a small shard of glass still caught in the raw flesh. My hand shakes a bit as I reach toward him with tweezers, but I can't afford to miss. "This might pinch. There is a piece of glass lodged in the wound."

"I'm sure I can take it," he says.

I place my left hand beneath his warm, rigid chin and focus on the shard while reaching toward it with the prongs of the tweezers. With a lungful of air holding me still, I pinch the metal clamps, thankful to have grasped it on the first try. The wound has a curved shape, making it hard to find the best direction to pull. The glass slides out with little force, but his jaw muscles tighten within my grip. "I'm sorry, Lieutenant."

"The sutures are ready," Audrey informs me.

"I doubt you'll need many. Seven or eight, if I have to take a guess."

"Would you laugh if I told you I've never had stitches before?" With a face like his, I can imagine he and his parents did what they could to protect such beauty, but I find his statement surprising for a man. Most boys find it to be a rite of passage into adulthood. There are too many trees to climb and rocks to scale.

"You've been lucky," I say. "I had to get stitches just once when I was around twelve or thirteen."

"What happened?" he asks, appearing intrigued—more intrigued than anyone else would sound while asking me this question.

"Yes, Lizzie, what happened? I've never heard this story," Audrey says.

"Oh, it was silly, really. I was roller skating down the street and a rock jumped out in front of me and took the lead."

"The rock won the race?" Everett asks.

"Twenty stitches on my right knee. It won all right."

"Fascinating," Audrey mutters. "It sounds like you did a fine job landing the aircraft with a broken gear."

I was avoiding the subject. The last thing Everett would want to focus on right now is what he just went through.

He winces at the pain from the needle before responding. "I should have double checked all the gears. It's my fault," he says through clenched teeth.

"Everyone is okay, and that's what matters," I follow.

"I need to go get some more dressing," Audrey says, breezing through the blue curtain.

"Go out with me tonight, Miss Salzberg. Please. I won't want to be alone with my thoughts after what happened today."

His question makes my heart quake. I know exactly what I

want to say in response, but the trouble it will cause forces me to pause. I narrow my eyes at Everett, marveling at the fact that he remembered my name, and his ability to be such a smooth talker. With such charming skills, it's hard not to wonder if he has a little black book full of women's names.

Without intention, I pinch my teeth against my bottom lip. "Lieutenant Anderson, are you aware of who my father is?"

The perplexing look in his glossy eyes tells me everything I have been questioning. "Should I?"

"Her father is Commander Douglas Salzberg," Audrey says, reentering the triage space. "He doesn't approve of Lizzie dating any man on this base."

The desire to smack my best friend for ratting me out is strong. I could have explained in a gentler way that didn't scare him off as fast.

"Ah, I see," Everett says. "You know I'm enlisted in the Army, not the Navy, correct?" Of course, I know this, but he might not understand how close the soldiers and sailors are that share this base. This island might be one of the larger Hawaiian Islands, but it's not that big.

"I do," I reply.

"Well, I don't see what the problem is?"

"Her father will kill you," Audrey says. "That would be the problem here." I nudge my shoulder into Audrey's. I understand she's trying to protect me from getting into a pickle, and maybe Everett from finding even more trouble here today, but I'm not getting any younger and a date with a Hollywood actor doesn't sound like the worst idea ever. Some girls would die to be in my shoes right now, maybe even Audrey.

"I'm happy to introduce myself to your father first and ask him if it's all right if you show me around town?" I'm willing to bet his thoughts are worse than Audrey's. "In fact, I insist on going about this in that way."

There goes that dream. "He won't go for the smooth talk or the charm," I assure him.

"Won't you let me at least try?" It's obvious he isn't giving up without a fight.

I complete the last of the sutures and tend to the bandages on his hands, hoping the wounds are not severe. "I thought you were trying to stay under the radar here," I suggest.

"Well, of course. And, I am, but a guy needs to have friends, right?"

"Friends?" I question.

"A guy would be pretty lucky to call a beautiful woman like you, a friend, don't you think?"

Maybe Dad wouldn't mind if I showed my new *friend* around base. I raise a brow. "You must be pretty confident in yourself to test the waters with my father, of all people."

Several minor cuts cover his knuckles, but nothing that requires sutures. "We can just clean these wounds and bandage them up. Then, you'll be as good as new, Lieutenant Anderson."

"Good. I'll have plenty of time to get home and shower before I come pick you up tonight. What do you say? Around six-thirty?"

My heart thuds like a meat cleaver banging against my ribcage. I don't want to get my hopes up, knowing Dad has no issues closing the door in someone's face. If we were to sneak around, we might have more of a chance at spending time together than if he does the "right thing" by asking Dad's permission, but with all eyes upon me, that wouldn't last long either.

"Good luck, Lieutenant. Mind if I watch how this plays out? I live just a few doors down?" Audrey states.

"By all means," Everett responds.

I lean back on my heels to peek out from behind the curtain to make sure the nurses aren't nearby as I break protocol by giving this man my address. "202 Lea Avenue," I whisper.

"Six-thirty," he says with a wink, a gesture I've seen on film many times. Women love his signature twinkling blink.

My cheeks burn at the thought of going out with him, forgetting about Dad for just a moment. It would be something else. "Sure," I say.

I secure the last bandage and drop my hands into my apron pockets.

"Thank you for your services here today. I appreciate the help."

"Anytime," Audrey says, waving as he walks away out of the small space between us.

"Did that just happen?" I ask, feeling breathless.

"Sign a handwritten death wish to your father? Yes, I believe you did," she says.

8

CURRENT DAY - OCTOBER 2018

KEIKI IS ARRANGING the pillows on my bed just inside the sliding glass doors. "Sweetheart, it's time for your afternoon nap," she calls out.

"I can come back another day," the man in front of me says. He's holding a notepad in his hand, gripping it so hard his hands are pale. I take a moment to study his face, wondering why I can't think of his name.

"Well—you've come all this way." The thought of being rude to this man makes me feel terrible.

"Gran, I live just down the street. It's no trouble at all."

An unexpected cough gums up my throat while I try to interpret the reason why this man is referring to me as his grandmother. Maybe he's confused or at the wrong house. "Down the street?" I question.

The man smiles, and a quiver in his lip shows a great deal of nerves. "Yes, Makena didn't want to be too far away, and you know how much she loves the beach just like you."

My granddaughter. They must be friends. *How nice.*

"Of course."

I glance inside at Keiki pulling down the covers on my bed. "Can I help you up?" the man asks, offering me his hand.

Without hesitation, I allow the man to help me to my feet and he guides me inside, embracing me as if I were a fragile piece of glass teetering at the edge of a tall shelf. I pass walls full of portraits, some constructed with oil paints, others with film. They make me smile and offer me a sense of warmth. "That man," I say, pointing at the grandest of hanging art, "I knew he was trouble from the very beginning."

"Is he the reason you couldn't date any of the men on base?" the man asks before I lower myself down onto the edge of my bed.

I stare into the perfect portrayal of his eyes painted with such detail. "No, he was not the reason. He was the lesson I had to learn."

"I've told you many times, love will blind you, Elizabeth. You are here to be a nurse. That must be your priority right now. You must save as many lives as possible. If you focus on your heart and your heartache, then those men in the room behind you will not make it," Dad said to me at a painstaking moment when I needed to hear that everything was going to be okay. I was desperate to know that love was not for nothing, and that it was worth fighting for.

"You don't understand, Dad," I said to him, as I stood on the blood-stained floors of the hospital while struggling to speak over the wails of pain. "I need to find him."

"Forget about that boy and go save some lives, Elizabeth. Do you hear me? You must be stronger than you think you are. Life does not reward us when we break."

I had never felt so much anger for Dad than I did in that moment, but it turned out he was right.

9

JULY 1941

WITH SLOW, long strokes from my hairbrush, I gaze out the window, trying to remember the last time I went on a date with a boy. Whatever dates I have been on, have been in secret because of the ridiculous rules Dad has in place. Maybe these rules haven't changed because Lewis and James don't bring any women home to meet Dad. I'm not sure if they are dating in secrecy or aren't interested in anyone on base, but it's never spoken about.

I can imagine the different scenarios of what might happen when Everett Anderson rings my doorbell, but I can't visualize a good ending. The arguments between Dad and me are useless. It's as if I'm talking to a wall when I try to reason with him. It's fair to say he's caused me to be secretive about my social life and extracurricular activities. I wonder if he thinks I'll never grow up enough to leave this house. If that is the case, it makes me feel sad for him. I don't want him to be alone for the rest of his life. Surely, Lewis and James will find wives and settle down. The guilt burns through me, but if I don't do what's best for me, no one will.

A knock on my door startles the ever-living daylights out of me, and I drop my hairbrush to the ground. "Elizabeth," Dad calls from the hallway. "Do you have a moment?"

He might wonder why I'm not in the kitchen waiting on the chicken casserole to finish baking. Any other night, I would have my eyes glued to a training manual on the countertop while I arrange side dishes for whatever I'm cooking. "Of course, Dad."

The door to my bedroom opens and Dad surveys me with a look of curiosity, as if he's trying to piece together an unsolvable mystery. I'm dressed in casual evening attire, my favorite red and white polka-dot tea dress, and the powder on my face is fresh. "Are you going somewhere?"

I stare into Dad's eyes for a long moment, debating my decision on how to carry out my plan. His matching hazel eyes to mine glisten below the hanging Tiffany's lamp above his head. There's something bothering him. I can see there's something swimming through his thoughts. He must sense I'm up to no good, not to his standards anyway. "Well, I'm going to the movie cinema with Audrey tonight. The casserole should be ready in about thirty minutes, though. I didn't want you three to go hungry."

"What are you girls planning to see? I didn't take notice of what was playing tonight?" he continues.

It's a good thing I took notice on my way home.

"Citizen Kane is showing tonight. I have been wanting to see it for some time and we are both free tonight." I could have left the last part out of my explanation. Audrey and I find ourselves bored silly most nights because we have little of a social life here on base.

"Citizen Kane, huh?" Dad responds. "I didn't think you would find interest in a murder mystery."

"Well, the picture is about the murder of a publisher. I find the plot to be intriguing."

"Good, I hope you enjoy it, then. Shall I expect you will be home before ten?"

He must know I'm too old for a curfew. As much as I want to tell him this again, it will lead me nowhere. "Of course." I glance at the bedside clock on my nightstand. I have less than fifteen minutes to figure out how to stop Everett from approaching my front door.

"Wonderful, I'm looking forward to hearing all about the movie when you return," Dad says, tipping his head before scanning the parameter of my bedroom as if looking for a clue to the lie he must be sure I'm telling. I snag my tube of lipstick and shove it into my purse. Dad reaches into his back pocket and pulls out a wad of cash, handing me a dollar bill. "I expect change."

"Yes, Dad, thank you."

His eyes narrow with a look of scrutiny, and my conscience is screaming inside my head. I hate lying, but he leaves me no choice. "I hope you boys enjoy supper."

"Yes, thank you for preparing the casserole. That was very thoughtful, especially since you're not joining us."

The moment Dad turns to leave my bedroom, I spritz my perfume on my neck and wrists, gather my shoes, and scurry to the front door. "Goodbye, Dad, I love you."

"Love you too, sweetheart," Dad says from his work desk.

I'm not sure where James and Lewis are, but I hope they aren't about to meet my presence on the street. That would be just my luck.

Once I'm outside, I draw in a sharp breath, fix my curls, and pull the lipstick and a compact out of my purse. While peering at the curve of my lashes through the reflection of my small mirror, a glare pulls my attention to the left. I spot a royal blue convertible Roadster cruising down the road. Gosh, if he is trying to stay under the radar, he isn't doing a good job. The gloss bouncing off his car has a more prominent reflection than my compact.

I trot down the sidewalk, waving my hands at him to stop a few houses down from mine. His dark aviator sunglasses prevent me from seeing whatever look might be in his eyes, but I suspect he's wondering what to do and likely curious why I'm not inside my house waiting on the doorbell to ring.

I open his passenger side door and plop into the seat. "Turn around in that driveway and go. Step on it!"

"Wait just a minute now. I promised to introduce myself to your father before we go out tonight. Miss Salzberg, I'm not a man who goes back on my word."

I purse my lips and smirk. "Lieutenant Anderson, I am certain you will have no chance at accompanying me anywhere tonight if you choose to meet my father." I can tell Everett isn't comfortable with this news, but he must decide, and be quick if he wants any hope of leaving here with me tonight.

"You are going to be a handful, aren't you?"

"Not as much as my father will be," I reply.

Relief fills my chest when Everett pulls the gear into reverse and backs into the nearest driveway. "Where shall I take you, miss troublemaker?"

I didn't think that far ahead. I figured someone would have caught us and stopped the car before turning off this street. "To the beach, just a few miles down the road." I'm not dressed in proper apparel for the beach, but it will be peaceful there at this time of day.

"The beach?" he questions.

"Do you trust me?" I reply.

"Absolutely not, Miss Salzberg." Everett takes a second to peer over at me with a mischievous smirk stretching toward his right dimple.

I interlace my fingers and rest my hands on my lap, trying my best to appear unaffected by every blink of his eyes. "Perfect. Let's go."

Everett doesn't make a peep until we are several streets away from where I live. "I don't feel right about this, Miss Salzberg."

"Elizabeth or Lizzie, but not Miss Salzberg, please," I say, scrunching my cheeks upward.

"Lizzie, I like that," he says, peering over at me through the corner of his eye. "If you don't mind me asking, why won't your father allow you to date? You must be at least eighteen, correct?"

It's embarrassing to admit I'm a twenty-year-old woman taking orders from my father the way I do. "I'm twenty and it's a long story. How old are you, Lieutenant?"

"Twenty-three, but I feel much older some days. Hollywood will do that to a man."

"I see, well, it can't be all that bad, living in the limelight."

Everett chuckles at my comment, but I was being serious. "I can honestly say the grass isn't always greener on the other side. I believe everyone has their burdens to bear."

"That could be true. I assume you don't get much privacy."

Everett's grip tightens around the white coated steering wheel and his jaw muscles flex. If there is anything I've mastered well, it's reading body language, and it's clear I have said too much.

"Would you mind telling me which way to turn? I'm still learning the roads here."

"Oh gosh, at the brick building on the right, take a left," I blurt out. "Sorry if I said too much. I tend to talk a lot—"

"You didn't say too much, Miss Salzberg—Lizzie."

"Take a right at the end of the street and you'll see a small parking area."

In silence we stroll down the two streets until we pull onto the fine gravel. "I didn't know there were multiple beaches on base."

"Most don't come here. It's small and the tide can be a pain sometimes."

Everett clamps his hands with a firm grip around the polished steering wheel. "I find it rather surprising that you aren't uncomfortable being here alone with me," he says.

It's hard to avoid the truth behind his comment, and I question if I've made a mistake by taking him here, but nothing has felt so right in such a long time. I place my finger against my lips to express my moment of contemplation. "I'm not sure I understand. Why would I be uncomfortable? Should I be?" Just because Dad doesn't trust another man on earth outside of our house shouldn't mean I must interrogate every gentleman I pass.

With slow movements, he lifts one hand from the steering wheel and brushes the back of his thumbnail against his bottom lip, highlighting the look of contemplation within his eyes. "You see, men from Hollywood, well, we often carry a reputation tied to our names."

The thought may have crossed my mind, but I see myself as an excellent judge of character, and I didn't feel a sense of unease either of the times we have run into each other. "No offense, Lieutenant Anderson, but you seem rather harmless to me."

"You shouldn't trust without a hitch, and please, call me Everett."

Maybe I should take notice of the warning signs he's offering or think twice about the decision I made tonight, but the only thing I feel is excitement bursting through my veins. The beach is a break from the reality of living on base. It's a place to contemplate, daydream, and listen to the wind's stories.

"You shouldn't be out with Commander Salzberg's daughter, but it looks like we're both taking some risks tonight, Everett."

While he makes his way around the front of his car toward my door, I comb my fingers through my hair to smooth out the mess from the humid air. I should have brought a scarf, but I was too eager to leave without making a peep that I forgot until we were halfway down the street.

Everett opens my door and offers me his hand. I'm glad I left my gloves behind too. His warmth sends a chill up my spine—the feeling is intoxicating. I lead him down a side path to the inlet of the beach where most people don't go because of the rocks. This area isn't safe for swimming because of the tide.

"I can't seem to figure you out, Lizzie." I slip my hand from his and climb up a couple stones to make myself comfortable.

"Why is that?"

"You aren't like anyone I've met. You don't care where I came from—who I was. Or so it seems. I can tell you are authentic and have a distinct mind of your own."

I straighten the pleats in my skirt to spill over my knees. "Well, to be fair, I was a big fan of yours on the big screen and I'm quite elated to have run into you here. However, the thought of dating has been so far from my mind that I didn't consider the idea of being here with you. Plus, you're different from everyone one else around here, and not just because you're famous. You're here for your noble reasons, and I'm intrigued."

Everett makes his way up the same couple of rocks and takes a seat beside me. He lifts his sunglasses from his face and folds them before sliding them into his shirt pocket. "I grew up with a silver spoon in my mouth—two parents involved in the entertainment industry, and a world full of illusions, or delusions. Everything I thought was normal was far from how most people live life. It makes me feel like an insignificant man—having life handed to me in such a way. I don't believe our journeys should be easy. I think we should be working toward making an impact and I don't believe I have done that by appearing on the big screen."

"That's absurd. Who cares if you grew up with more money

than others? You have entertained this country. How can you not consider that to be an impact?"

"Anyone can entertain, but I'm capable of more, Lizzie. I have something to prove to myself and it's more than being able to perform in front of a camera."

I stifle a laugh, not intending for it to be at him but alongside him. To feel similar but in a different way makes our rendezvous seem like destiny. "Just as you might think many wouldn't understand you, I don't feel understood either. I want to see the world, but not by lavish means. I want to be on the front lines with our men and take care of our country in a way that makes me feel like I've done something worthwhile. My mom was the same way and I feel the need to carry on her legacy and see it through because she couldn't. I believe it's my path. Then, when the war is over, I want to travel to see all the wonders of the world. I want to swim in the Dead Sea, walk the Great Wall of China, explore the Egyptian pyramids. And maybe, I'll be lucky enough to see what's on the other side of the clouds up there."

"The clouds?" Everett chuckles.

"Yes, the clouds—I think there is a reflection of our world up there—another side we know nothing about," I say, refusing to shy away from my illusionary thoughts.

"I'd happily fly you through the clouds if you want to explore," he says with a smirk.

"I won't forget you said this," I say, nudging my shoulder against his.

"Good. But first, you will be a nurse. That's where your adventure starts, right?" he asks.

"Yes, but in truth, I desire to join the Army Nurse Corps, but my father won't allow me to do such a thing." I twist my head to witness the expressive response to my comment, but Everett's eyes lock on the horizon as if he's baffled by my desire.

"The world is at war. It's a brutal time to join the Army, but I believe if someone is eager to step forward and be a brave face in front of the enemy, it's his calling. The stories I've heard from Europe, though, they haunt me in my sleep. I enlisted just over a year ago, and to see the wreckage of what has occurred in such a short time is daunting. I can only hope the United States remains neutral and out of the battle zone."

Our conversation isn't what I expected it to be tonight. I somewhat assumed he would be pursuing me with wooing words while staring into my eyes as if I was a piece of candy ready to melt in his hand, but I was wrong.

"Whatever might happen is unforeseeable, but I'm not basing the point of my compass off fear. I want to be a nurse and aid in any way I can. For now, that means from the hospital here on base, but it's something, I suppose."

"Don't degrade your purpose, Lizzie. I needed you today, and you were there to put me back together."

"And I'm glad I was there."

"Say, how about a bite to eat downtown? I'm starving right now."

Downtown. A place where everyone will see me and know who I'm with, and I forgot my darn scarf.

10

JULY 1941

WITH MY HAND shielding the side of my face as Everett and I stroll back to the car, it's clear I'm more concerned about someone seeing us than he is, but I'm the one who must encounter my father when I go home tonight. It's completely absurd. I'm treated like a child, but I am falling right into the trap by acting as one. This could be the highlight of my life and may likely be the turning point that forces me to put my foot down and stand firm to Dad.

After we make our way back to the car, I notice a contemplative look in Everett's eyes. He looks like he's trying to figure something out, but I'm not sure what.

"I'm intrigued to hear why your father has such a firm dismay for you dating. I'm sure no father is ready to let his daughter move on with her life, but I imagine he wants you to find happiness and someone to share your life with."

After all these years of living on base, I'm not sure I've had an encounter with a man so forward; one who speaks such strong thoughts out loud.

"I bet I know why," he continues without allowing me a long enough moment to conjure a sensible reply to a nonsensical topic.

I suppose I would rather buy some time and allow him to guess at Dad's reasons for always keeping a hawk's eye on me.

"What is your guess, Everett?" Maybe his assumption will enlighten me.

Everett slouches into his seat and relaxes his elbow on the window frame and his other hand on the wheel. "I bet you had a rotten experience with some fella here on base and your father can't bear the thought of seeing your heart broken again."

The story seems logical. Any other narrative would be too heavy for a casual night out. I offer a smile to respond without lying. "It sounds like you've seen a thing or two."

"I've seen a few broken hearts, and I've had some scripts that had me acting like I had one myself, but in all honesty, I haven't experienced it firsthand. From what I've seen, I think I'd rather spare myself that type of pain."

"I can only imagine how many hearts you have broken, unknowingly of course," I suggest, batting my lashes through a peep out of the corner of my eyes.

Everett slaps his left hand down to his knee. "Now, that's unfair of you to assume. I have broken no one's heart. If I'm not mistaken, a girl would need to share her heart with me for that to happen."

I find his words hard to believe. Girls fan themselves at the mere mention of his name, so I can only imagine how many women would pay money to be sitting in this car with him right this second.

Everett finds his way to the center of town and spots a prime parking spot in front of the strip of restaurants we can choose from. He slides his sunglasses back on and straightens the collar of his pressed shirt. As he did earlier, he opens my door and offers his hand. Currents of nerves run with vigor through my blood as I imagine the look on each face we pass. I'm not sure who wouldn't recognize him, even with sunglasses. He may think there are only a few people who know he's living here now, but word has spread like a raging fire. It has been the highlight of chatter in every corridor in the hospital, the break room, training room, and even triage. I'm not sure how long he thinks his presence will go unnoticed.

"What's good here? I've only been to the chow hall since arriving."

"Well, what type of food do you prefer?" I ask, feeling his hand settle on my back as I take the lead.

"Authentic. I've been dying to taste the flavors of the island." I hate to be the bearer of bad news, but what he might consider authentic here on base can't compare to some smaller restaurants across remote areas of Oahu. However, if he hasn't tried elsewhere, he won't have anything to compare the food to, I suppose.

"If you enjoy seafood, you may like Honi Makai," I say, pointing down the block.

"I do, very much so."

For someone who could gain attention from anyone he desires, he's quite laid back and easygoing. If I hadn't seen him on the big screen with my own eyes, I wouldn't be thinking past his appeal and poise. Instead, I'm bubbling at the mouth with questions about what it's like to live as a movie star.

Honi Makai is rather empty, likely because of the film playing in the theatre next door—the precise location of where I am claiming to be. A few lingering looks from people passing by make me wonder if someone might say something to him. Maybe they aren't sure he's Everett Anderson, or they can't figure out why on earth, of all people on this base, he would be out with Commander Salzberg's daughter.

We're seated at a small table toward the back of the restaurant, but against the wall-length window separating us from the sidewalk. Everett doesn't lift his menu right away. Instead, he fixes his eyes on me, staring with a piercing inflection of wonder. "I'm not sure why I feel like I have known you much longer than a measly week. There's something about you that feels familiar."

"Is this another infamous line, Everett Anderson?" The flattery is hard to hide with how warm my cheeks feel, but I'm determined to figure out why this man would want to spend an evening with me. Any nurse could have fixed the wound on his temple today. Beyond that, who would find themselves attracted to the klutz of a girl knocking over shelves and a Spam display at the commissary?

He doesn't seem offended or appalled by my question. Instead, he appears to stare harder, deeper into my eyes as if he's trying to see my soul. I break our stare because the heat within me is almost too much to bear. My heart pounds and I refuse to be a fool for seeing tonight as anything more than a chance to say I went on a date with The Everett Anderson.

"Have you lived on Oahu your entire life?" he asks.

"I have. My father's commitment to the Navy is for life and has been since he turned eighteen."

"And your mother?"

It's been a while since I've had to respond to this question. Mostly anyone I cross paths with knows all there is to know about Mom so when the topic arises, my body stiffens, I lift my chin, and swallow the knot forming in my throat. "She passed away five years ago from polio."

This is the part where people bow their head and change the sound of their voice to emit sympathy while offering condolences. "I lost my mother, as well. It's been seven years. She suffered from melancholia until it took her life one night while my father and I were out to dinner." My eyes grow wide while taking in his statement. I don't know of anyone who has done something so awful. The thought of a mother making a choice to end her life is unfathomable. I can't imagine how much this must have affected him. The blame he must carry around, that he wasn't there to stop her, is terrible.

There was a time when I blamed Mom for the way she died, even though the disease wasn't in anyone's control. Though, in some ways, I often thought she was asking to contract the disease when volunteering to help with polio outbreaks. As the years passed, I let go of those thoughts, finding them tied to grief.

Everett doesn't seem to have found a way of coping with his mother's death, so he just speaks about it matter-of-factly.

The lump in my throat is hard to swallow as I try to think of proper words to respond, but what is a person to say in this situation?

The quiet between us is painstaking as we digest each other's woes. I wouldn't wish this shared anguish on anyone.

"Okay, what do you do for fun, Lizzie?" Everett changes the subject as if a clapperboard has motioned an action.

"For fun?" I repeat his question, stalling with an answer.

"Yes, you know ... what makes you smile?"

It isn't purposeful or preventable when a grin curls along my lips.

Everett's face brightens to a light shade of red and he places his finger above his top lip as if embarrassed to be a reason I smile. "I enjoy writing and exploring."

"You don't say?" His jaw falls open, masking the blush along his cheeks. "Where do you like to explore?"

"Everywhere and anywhere. Sometimes, I go where the wind takes me. I never know what I'll stumble across. It can be quite exciting."

"Maybe I could join you on one of your wandering adventures. There must be a lot of hidden stunning landscapes to uncover here on the island."

I glance out the window toward the small view of the ocean we have between the storefronts on the other side of the street. "I'm not sure I'll make a wonderful teacher, but I could try." Of course, I must figure out alternative ways to sneak out of my house and stay out of the public eye.

I lift my menu after spotting a look from one server who I suspect is waiting to take our order. Everett follows my lead but chooses the first item his eyes stop at.

"Mahi Mahi?" I question.

"How did you know?"

"You're not a local just yet," I jest.

"I better work on that. What about you? What are you going to have?"

I press my lips together and grin. "I'll have the same, so you aren't eating Mahi Mahi alone."

"So I don't look like the new guy on base, you mean?"

"I didn't say any such thing."

The server notices as we place our menus down and tends to the table. "We'll both have the Mahi Mahi," Everett says, making it known that the Hawaiian language is as foreign to him as the fish.

"Mahalo," I offer my gratitude to the server as she collects our menus.

"Mahalo. Right. I keep forgetting. That means, hello, goodbye, and thank you, right?"

"Kind of, but not always. Mahalo is a way to show appreciation, but also, some people feel grateful to be around others and will use the word as a greeting too."

"Well, mahalo, little sis."

I didn't see James walk inside the restaurant. I didn't think he would be downtown tonight. He never goes out on the weekends, never mind a Friday night. Now, I'm the one with my jaw hanging ajar. Everett shoots up from his chair, ready to salute James. "What are you doing here?"

"Me?" he questions, as if I shouldn't be at liberty to question my brother. "I was out to meet a friend for ice cream and saw you while walking by the window here. Surely, you can understand why I'm confused since Dad told me you were at the movies with Audrey. I should have figured something was up when I saw her outside watering the flowers when I left the house. You should tell her she isn't an excellent cover story. Or did you forget to tell her about the lie?"

"Thank you, James. Well, I think you should continue on to the ice cream shop so you aren't late for whoever you are meeting there."

I know James won't walk away without taking a moment to introduce himself to Everett. I'm not sure he knows who Everett is since he doesn't pay attention to the movies or celebrity news, but I'm about to find out.

"Lieutenant Everett Anderson. It's a pleasure to meet you, Sir." He's calling James a sir. This is just perfect. James will let that go right to his head.

"No kidding," James says. "No wonder you snuck out."

"James," I say, gritting my teeth.

"Don't worry, sis. Your secret is safe with your big brother. I wouldn't rat you out."

James takes a step in toward Everett and drops his hand on his shoulder, whispering something into his ear. I can't hear what he is saying, but by the look on Everett's face, I assume it involves a threat of some form.

"I have no intentions of keeping your sister out late," Everett says in response to the secret.

"Great. Well, I hope you enjoy your meals. I'm going to enjoy my ice cream, and we will chat more about this little rendezvous later." James's smile is making my stomach hurt. I know he won't rat me out, but it doesn't mean he won't take advantage of holding something over my head. Certain things in our family will never change, no matter how old we all get.

"I shouldn't have let you run off with me before meeting your father," Everett says as soon as James walks out of the restaurant. He can't take the blame for this after having intentions of doing the right thing by me. I knew how it would end and I wanted to go out with him tonight.

"This isn't your fault and James *is all talk*. He won't tell my father a word about this. You don't have to worry. My brothers are the only two on base who protect me from my father as much as my father protects me from everyone else."

"Brothers, as in multiple," Everett repeats, with a nervous chuckle.

I wonder if he's going to get up and run now or wait until after we eat our Mahi Mahi.

11

JULY 1941

JAMES MIGHT NOT BE HOME YET. That would be the best case. The movie won't be over for another twenty minutes and if we continue driving on this road, I will be home a half hour too early. Dad will know I made up a story. I suppose I could come clean and fight the fight by arguing that he must stop telling me what I can do at twenty years old. Then, he'll remind me he still pays for the roof I live under and that I can't support myself, nor will anyone else, and therefore, he has a right to dictate the rules. I could duel him on the subject until our last breaths, but I believe I inherited his stubbornness.

"What are you going to do about your situation?" Everett asks. It's a question I ponder every morning as I wonder why my life mimics one that would go along with somebody that's in love and married. The way my life is unfolding isn't what I want.

"There are three months left of class before I earn my certification. Once that happens, I plan to secure a full-time job and see where life takes me." There isn't a response that explains my intent to walk away from the life of a teenage girl playing the role of a housewife. "The idealism of supporting myself is a dream. Traveling and exploring the world is a fantasy. But, finding a man to settle down with is just what it sounds like—settling. I'm not sure I want to slow down and move on to a place of complacency. This may sound crazy and unnatural, but I have a desire to live life to the fullest. I prefer to die while experiencing the wonders of the world rather than end up falling asleep in a rocking chair and never waking up again."

We're at one of the few stop signs in the area without another headlight in sight. Everett twists his neck to glance over, the shimmer in his eyes capturing the illumination of a nearby gas lamp.

"There is no worse feeling than settling for less than what you deserve," he says.

Coming from the mouth that ate off a silver spoon, it seems one of us might view this topic in a different light.

"Men and women have a predetermined path in life. There are paths rockier than others: some lined with red carpets, others have forks in the road. There's no roadmap to tell us which way to go in life, so we must follow our hearts. What else can we trust?"

His words soothe me like warm honey, making me believe there's hope for more than what's laid out in front of me. I don't want the thought of adventure to be a dream. "What are you saying, Lieutenant Anderson?" I ask, leaning in toward him with a desire for more of his enlightening thoughts.

Everett takes my hand from the leather upholstery of my seat and weaves his fingers between mine. Warmth fills my chest and melts down the center of my core. "I'm saying, let nothing impede your desires or dreams. This is your life, and you are in control of your destiny."

He lifts my knuckles to his lips and lowers our clasped hands back to the seat. His foot eases onto the gas pedal and we cruise in silence, driving toward a different direction rather than my house. "The movie doesn't end for a few minutes. I think it might be okay to get a little lost on the way back to your street. I might not be in favor of supporting lies to your father, but I support you doing what makes you happy."

"Pull up over there," I say, pointing up the road to an outer bank ledge.

"Yes, Ma'am." The crackling of the rocks beneath the tires offers me a sense of calm, knowing I can stall a little longer before going home. The cliff overlooks the ocean, revealing an ethereal-looking reflection of deep blues and teals that complement the surrounding greenery of the mountains and starlit sky. "Do you ever tire of the view?"

"Never. As a child, I dreamed of growing up to be a mermaid. It was a sad day when I learned the truth about the mystical sea princesses."

Everett chuckles and scratches his fingertips along the side of his face. "I think it's sweet to have an ambitious life goal at a young age."

"You are kindly trying to tell me that I'm adorable," I correct him.

"No, I mean it. I had no plans aside from acting because it is what my parents decided they wanted me to do."

"They think they know everything, I suppose."

"Well, I guess we're showing them they're wrong."

"You have," I say. "I'm still living at home answering to my father."

"But in a few months, that will all change. You'll be free to go wherever you want and do as you please," he says, reminding me of my words.

"Maybe I should send you out with my friend, Audrey, next time. There's no sense in wasting time with a disoriented girl like me, is there?"

Everett shifts around in his seat to face me. "Well, wait just a darn minute, Miss Lizzie. Here I am, thinking we had a wonderful night, and I am, seconds away from asking you out on a second date. Why in the world would I want to go out with one of your friends?"

I'm embarrassed by my assumption but speaking about the thought of running off into the unknown in a few months doesn't paint an ideal picture for our potential future. "Well, I figured since you are so understanding of my passionate desires to run away, you might not want to spend time around a girl without a plan."

"Lizzie, my plan is to not have one at all. Life will happen as it should. I'd like to see you again, and if it's something you might enjoy too, I won't give your lack of intention a second thought. I'm alive right now, in this moment, and it's a pretty darn wonderful moment if you ask me."

"You talk in circles, you know that?"

"Does it make you dizzy?" His words lower in volume and a slow smile curls along his lips.

"Very much so."

"Well, good. It's time to get you home now. The movie just ended."

"What an ending," I say as a shiver tingles up my spine.

"And maybe ... it's the beginning of something new," he replies.

The stars sparkle into a blur as I rest the back of my head against Everett's outstretched arm while we continue down the quiet streets of my neighborhood. One little white lie for a night like tonight could become a mess of many tall tales.

"You can stop right over there at the corner."

"Lizzie, you must not be serious. Your house is at least five or six houses away from the corner."

"Six, yes, but my dad is home and if he spots your car—well, it will put a damper on this remarkable night."

"Gosh, you are making this complicated. I'm going to watch you walk home, if that's all right? I'll feel better knowing you are inside safely."

"Of course, but I'll have you know I've walked home from Audrey's house many times this late at night. I assure you there's no need to worry."

"I understand," he says, pulling up along the corner. He reaches for his door handle. I assume he is planning to open my door, but there's no need if he isn't joining me on my walk. I place my hand on his, the one resting on the steering wheel. "Everett, thank you for a lovely evening. I had a swell time."

"May I get the door for you?"

I try to suppress the giggle working up through my chest, but it slips out. "You are incredible and sweet, but I'm the type of girl who is happy to open a door on her own."

Everett dips his head, almost as if he must collect his thoughts. "Well, Miss Lizzie, I am the type of man who insists on opening doors for ladies, so I'm not sure how this could affect our future dates, but I hope you'll come around to the idea of letting a man treat you as special as you are." The slight smirk teasing one side of his lips shows his humor, but I sense there is more than a little truth to his statement.

"Well, next time, keep the car rolling and I'll jump right on out. How about that?"

"Trouble. You are a handful. I guess I was right to assume so earlier tonight. Nevertheless, I find you terribly fascinating. Plus, I believe you just said there will be a next time, so does that mean we can do this again?"

"If it is up to me, yes, but if you come to realize I'm too much trouble for you, I understand, Lieutenant Anderson." I blow him a kiss from the palm of my hand and push the passenger door open just enough to slip out onto the street. "Good night, now."

"Good night, doll-face."

I spin on my heels, reminding myself of my distaste for that name, doll-face, but for some ridiculous reason, hearing it from his mouth makes my heart skip a beat. It's obvious I'm not as tough as I thought. I can't even fan myself off as I walk down the row of houses because I have yet to hear the motor of his car ignite. He's watching me until I make it home. It's a sweet gesture. He isn't like the boys I have snuck around with before. Everett is by far the truest definition of a gentleman.

I'm not sure he can see the small wave I offer before opening the front door to my house, but I'm certain he can't see the smile on my face. Dad, however, will be much too aware of the look on my face. I pull in a deep breath, relax my shoulders and rush through the door, swinging around as usual while hanging my pocketbook up on the coat hook. "How was the casserole?" I ask, noticing the sleepy look in his eyes.

"Supper was great. Thank you, Elizabeth. How was the picture?"

I turn back for my bag, retrieving the dollar he gave me before I left the house. I don't have change to show I spent the quarter. My eyes widen as I try to think of a quick reason. "The theatre was having some difficulties with the film and it had to restart several times. It was quite a nuisance, so we were all given our money back." I turn to face Dad with the dollar bill.

"You didn't stop to have a bite to eat? I figured you and Audrey would have a snack at least."

"Oh, you know we made a silly bet, and she owed me a coke and a popcorn, so she paid tonight. I guess it was just a lucky night." Dad is looking at me with speculation and a raised brow. "The theatre didn't give you twenty-five cents back when they refunded you?"

"Well, of course not. They were counting out the seventy-five cents, but I handed them change I already had and took the dollar instead. It's much easier to carry than a handful of coins. Right?" I'm no stranger to making up stories on the spot, and by the look on Dad's face, my response comes quick enough to satisfy his curiosity.

"You're a smart girl, Elizabeth. Good thinking, sweetheart."

"What can I say? I'm a chip off the old block." I might take my act a little too far sometimes. "Well, I'm off to bed now. Sweet dreams."

"Goodnight, Elizabeth." Dad clears his throat and releases a groan as he leans back into the old sofa. I assume he will sit there for the next hour speculating on the different ways I might fib about my night, but if James doesn't make a peep, I think I have my bases well covered this time.

12

CURRENT DAY - OCTOBER 2018

WHEN I OPEN my eyes to find the sun in the middle of the sky outside my window, I realize it's the middle of the day rather than first thing in the morning. I hate naps. It's something children take so they don't become cranky by mid-afternoon. Plus, it means I must recapture every thought I held clearly in my mind before falling asleep. Another clean slate with nothing but empty walls where memories used to hang. "How was your nap, sweetheart?" Keiki asks from the chair next to my bed.

"Well, I don't quite remember, but I suppose it was just like any other nap," I say with a grin.

"I can imagine," Keiki says with a soft laugh. "Daniel left for a bit. I thought you may have exhausted yourself from answering his questions."

I push myself up on the bed to lean upright against my pillow. "Daniel?"

"Yes, dear, Makena's husband, he was here to pick your brain about Pearl Harbor for an article he's writing."

"I thought I was dreaming about that," I say with a sigh. "Keiki, would you be a darling and find my journal? I believe I left it out on the — out there," I say, pointing outside.

Keiki hurries outside and retrieves my leather-bound journal and hands it to me. "Is everything okay?"

"Yes, it's just that sometimes I leave notes in here for myself so I can remember what happened earlier in the day."

Keiki places her hand down on top of the leather. "Sweetheart, I don't think you've written anything in that book for quite some time now."

I look up at her worrisome eyes, wondering how she could know such a thing. "Oh, don't be silly, I write all my greatest memories in this book. See, I'll show you." I open the flap and fan through the first several dozen pages. "Ah, here, this is recent. I wrote about those beautiful birds I see every morning."

I press my finger to the ashen page and read the words aloud.

After the white birds with red wings filled the sky, everything has changed. There is darkness at night, nothing but the stars and moonlight glistening against the rippling waters. Streetlights are merely for decoration rather than use, and electricity is something we can only appreciate during the daylight hours. The grocery lists are shorter, our suppers less filling. We're learning to appreciate what we once had, and it's a lesson we must have needed. To have nothing feels as though we once had it all.

Sirens sing in the night, sometimes in the morning, but when the call goes out, we secure our gas masks as quickly as we can. It's for practice to expect the unexpected. The rubber seal will protect us from a poison gas attack and offer the ability to inhale purified air, but the clunky canister hanging from my face makes me feel like I'm suffocating. My skin becomes damp and itchy, and it's hard to see through the dark eye holes. It's a daily reminder of the danger we cannot escape and losing the freedom this country has fought so hard for.

— DECEMBER 21, 1941

"How about some tea? Would you like that?" Keiki asks as I reach the end of the page I was reading.

"Maybe this passage isn't new," I digress. "I can clearly recall that time when we had to follow so many rules and live like we were in the dark ages at night. What a year that was—I truly did not know what was to come. I was more concerned about being caught in a forbidden romance than an earth-shattering change to our world."

With a gentle tug, Keiki takes the journal from my hands and places it on my nightstand. "Sweetheart, I'm going to go put the tea kettle on the stove. Maybe you could watch some television for a few minutes. It's just about time for *Young and the Restless*, your favorite," she says, handing me the remote control.

It's humorous to think I spend my late days watching soap operas. The beloved pastime of listening to these dramas on the radio was the thing to do as a woman in the forties, but it wasn't for me because I did not want to adhere to the ways of a housewife. It was the last thing on my mind, but being swept off my feet by a dreamboat—that's another story. Those are the memories I enjoy replaying in my mind's eye over and over.

13

JULY 1941

IT'S BEEN a full week since the evening I spent with Everett. My delusion of stumbling upon him somewhere on base hasn't happened. There was no way I could give him my phone number, knowing the likelihood of Dad answering the call. I was in such a fog that night; I assumed we would just find each other again. However, I do not know where he might be during any hour of the day. I'm sure his schedule is much like James and Lewis's, moving from location to location tending to different tasks and duties throughout the day. Of course, I should be thankful he hasn't shown up at the hospital since I don't wish to see him in those circumstances again. However, being the nurse who sutured the wound on Everett's temple, I know it's been a week's time and he needs to have the sutures removed. Of course, I'm not a nurse on staff and for all I know he could have been here, had them removed and I wouldn't be any wiser of his visit.

"Your face is going to get stuck like that if you don't start blinking again," Audrey whispers from the seat next to mine. "Plus, you'll have a red splotch on your cheek all day from leaning on your hand. What could be so important to make you look like a tired ghoul?"

"It's been a long week," I say.

Audrey intertwines her fingers, folding them on top of her open book. "Lizzie, I warned you he was a bad idea."

"If you'd please open your textbooks to page two-forty, we'll begin there," Nurse Jones instructs us.

Audrey and I both flip through the pages of our book. "He is not a bad idea. He's indeed quite a wonderful idea," I argue.

"We have three months left, Lizzie. You must keep your head from floating in the clouds. He's a soldier with the Army Air Corps of all jobs. There is no way he has time to track you down." I know she's correct in what she's saying, but no one can stop me from daydreaming.

The remaining hours of the day crawl by and I become dizzy while I stare at the red second hand on the clock. The last three months of our training comprise of nothing more than reviews on everything we've learned over the last few years. I'm certain I haven't forgotten a thing, and I'm bored silly listening to the rookie topics.

"Okay, ladies, I will see you bright and early tomorrow. Don't forget to review the chart on seizure and symptoms. I will quiz you tomorrow."

I toss my bookmark between the pages we left off on and slap the cover shut.

"Do you have somewhere to be?" Audrey asks as I drop my book and notepad into my satchel.

"No, not at all, why do you ask?"

She spends a moment longer, making room in her bag for her belongings. "I haven't seen you move this fast in a while."

"I just need some fresh air, is all." Being cooped up in this room all day causes me to crave the warmth of the sun on my shoulders and a chance to breathe in the scent of flowers rather than cleaning agents.

I stand from my seat, tapping my toe with eagerness while waiting for Audrey to follow. It's almost as if she's trying to slow me down.

"Are you feeling okay?" she asks.

"Yes, yes, why?"

"My goodness. You're making me feel like I need air." Audrey says, rising from her seat and draping her satchel over her shoulder.

I take the lead out into the corridor, keeping my eyes set on the sun shining through the front entrance. The moment I step outside, the fresh air calms my nerves. "It's so stuffy in there sometimes," I say to Audrey.

"I don't know if I would call the air inside stuffy with the amount of ammonia the cleaning staff uses, but I can see how you might enjoy the outdoors more."

Anytime I'm outside, I can't help myself from glancing around the area, looking for a glimpse of Everett. I think I'm going bonkers. A man has never gotten me all worked up before. This isn't like me. "I was thinking of stopping at the dress shop on the way home. Are you interested in joining me?" I ask Audrey.

She peers down at her wristwatch. "Sure, I have about an hour to spare. Are you shopping for anything special or do you just want to peruse the racks?"

"Yes, that," I say, still searching the area.

"Lizzie, come over here for a moment." Audrey lifts her satchel from her shoulder and takes a seat on the short stone wall to the side of the walkway.

I take the few steps over to her and lower my satchel to place beside hers. "What is it you want to talk about?"

Her eyes speak before her mouth. Her brows curl in toward one another and her lips twist to the side. "Sweetie, I'm worried about you. I can see the sparkles glistening in your eyes, even after an entire week has gone by, and I don't want to see you get hurt."

"You have goals and dreams of joining the Army Nurse Corps and you know we can't do so unless we're unmarried. I'm just wondering what the point to all of this is if it can't go any further?"

The question feels accusatory, and I hate to be reminded of silly rules. I cross my arms over my chest, feeling like I must defend myself. "Well, first, my father has forbidden me from joining the Army Nurse Corps. Therefore, I shouldn't concern myself with the Army's rule, correct? And if I'm not mistaken, women get married so they can start a family, have children. Since raising a family is quite far from my mind, there isn't a need to get married despite my feelings for someone. The Army wouldn't be able to tell me who I can love. Therefore, if I chose to enlist, being unwed is not an issue I need to be concerned with, right?"

"When did you decide to follow your father's wishes? I thought you were still contemplating the Army Nurse Corps?"

I have gone back and forth on my thoughts many times, but a plan requires me to know what will happen weeks or months from now, and I'm not interested in thinking that far ahead. Life might take me in a completely different direction for all I know. "Well, who knows what will happen three months from now. I will not live as if I'm dying tomorrow. That's absurd."

"Your vision is blurry, Lizzie. These words don't even sound as if they are your own. What has happened to you?"

I don't have an answer because I see nothing wrong with what I'm saying. It's true, neither of us knows what the future holds. Why should I make so many assumptions when nothing in life has ever gone as planned? My gaze drifts up toward the clouds in the sky, taking inventory of the shapes and patterns. A mere look into the blue oblivion will set my thoughts free, like a clenched fist releasing the string of a weightless balloon. Mom would often tell me this when upset over fickle things.

"Well, if you ask me, I say it looks like a flying elephant."

I lower my head at the sound of a voice different from Audrey's. First, I see my very best friend tenting her fingers on her forehead. I turn toward a voice that jolts my heart, finding another set of eyes gazing into the sky alongside me. "Everett," I say, sounding more enthusiastic than I should reveal after one date. My cheeks burn in response to his dimpled smile.

"You are a hard woman to track down."

"That's because her father is Commander Salzberg," Audrey replies before I find the right words to respond with.

"Audrey, right?" Everett offers his hand to her. "It's lovely to see you again."

I'm surprised to see Audrey shake his hand and respond with a smile. "I'm sure Lizzie feels the same about you," she responds.

"Pardon me if I'm interrupting you, ladies. It's not my intention." There isn't a need to feel that way, but Audrey is making this encounter far more intense than it needs to be.

"Don't be silly," Audrey says. "In fact, I was just about to find my bicycle. Lizzie, will you be joining me or—"

It's as if I've forgotten how to speak or lost my tongue as I look between Audrey and Everett. "I—well—"

"Would you mind if I steal your friend for an hour?" Everett asks Audrey.

I can hear the word, yes, without her so much as uttering a peep. "Of course not. By all means, see if you can't do something about this girl with her head lost in the clouds."

I shoot Audrey a disagreeing look, wondering why she's being so rude to Everett and embarrassing me at the same time. "I wish you would listen to me," she mutters while leaning in for a hug. "Please protect your heart, Lizzie. You're my best friend and I can't bear to witness you go through any more pain than you've already been through."

I squeeze her arms a little tighter than necessary. "I will be just fine. No need to worry, sweetie."

"All right, then. Maybe I'll stop by after dinner for some tea."

"That sounds wonderful. I'll see you then."

"Everett, I hope you have a pleasant night," she says, hopping down from the wall with her bag.

Neither of us speak until Audrey is out of sight. "Did I say something to upset her?" Everett asks.

"Oh, no. It's not that."

"Gosh. Then, what is it?"

"It's nothing, I promise."

Everett inhales a lungful of the floral filled air. "Well, then. Today is the first day I haven't had training at this hour, and I thought I might catch you leaving class."

I take my satchel from the wall and place it over my shoulder. "I suppose I didn't think about how hard it might be to run into each other again. Although it looks as if you still haven't had those sutures removed."

"You said seven to ten days, if I'm not mistaken," he responds.

"Most people show up on the seventh day."

"Well, truth be told, I've become quite attached to them."

His words take a quick moment to resonate when I realize the humor within his response. I place the back of my hand against my mouth, trying to suppress a heavier laugh than a lady should offer this man. "You're quite comical."

"What can I say? I was sure I would have you in stitches with laughter by now."

This time I feel caught off-guard and can't control the laughter rumbling through me. "Well, you are something else, Lieutenant Anderson — Everett."

"Say, could I persuade you to take a stroll to the park? I'd love to spend a little time with you."

"I'd enjoy that very much."

Everett slips his fingers beneath the strap of my satchel and takes it from my grip. "Allow me."

He doesn't place the straps over his shoulder. He couldn't, not in his starched and pressed dress pinks. In this heat, he'd have a permanent crease where he shouldn't have one.

As we're walking side by side, I reach for his left hand to inspect the damage from last week, seeing the minor cuts have healed up well. "Your hand looks much better."

"It is quite nice looking, isn't it?" he says, inspecting the pink marks left behind.

"I didn't realize you were such a jokester last week."

"Life without humor is like a pie with no filling. What's the use?"

I press my lips together into a stifled smile. "Goodness, you are on a roll."

"Just buttering you up, I suppose."

I flap my hand against his arm. "You are bad, you know that?"

"I do, but in all seriousness, miss Lizzie, I was hoping to see if you would like to join me for another evening on the town? Of course, I'm more than happy to speak to your father first, but I respect your feelings on the matter too."

The small park full of greenery and wooden benches peeks over the hill. As usual, the area is quite empty except for a couple of mothers with baby carriages taking their afternoon walks. "I would love to go out again, but I'm afraid it still will not be following my father's permission."

"Understood. Could I take you somewhere outside the base?"

"I'd like that." No watchful stares or brothers looming around the corner.

We stop between a cluster of thick nut trees bordering the grassy area of the park. The shade lowers the temperature a few degrees, offering a welcome relief from July's unforgiving sun. "Is it my former status your friend Audrey doesn't like?"

I didn't realize he was still hanging onto Audrey's words or attitude, but I might be too if one of his friends spoke to me the way she had. It's unlike her to be so protective or concerned for my well-being. She has no problem telling me what's what when I'm looking for an escape she might not agree with, but I merely run off for an afternoon trip to the beach. It's hardly something to get in a tizzy about. In fact, sometimes I feel like she's siding with Dad in a way. It's maddening.

"Oh, no. Of course not. Audrey doesn't condone lying or withholding information like I am with my father. She's also mentioned the required status of an Army Nurse needing to be unwed. It's all a bunch of horse feathers if you ask me."

"Well, she has a good point, but why worry about marriage when you might despise me come a month from now?"

"That was my exact thought. It's as if you can read my mind," I jest with him. "My father won't change his mind on the matter, and there's no use in arguing my point to him. Therefore, I plan to live the way I see fit and if someone would like to join me on my path to wherever I'm going, it would be splendid."

"If I'm being honest, I have been searching through crowds downtown every night for the past week. I needed to find you. I'm quite fond of the way your mind works. It's alluring to see a woman seeking her desires without fearing obstacles."

"Alluring?" I repeat, lifting my brows in response. Then, I peer down to my feet after hearing the word form on my tongue. Alluring. I don't think anyone has ever said this to me.

Everett slips his finger beneath my chin and with a gentle nudge, redirects the view of my stare up into his eyes. "And beautiful. Stunning, without a doubt. But inside—you're magnificent, like a hypnotic melody that blacks out the world around me from anything more than your existence." As if instinctual, my hand draws into my chest, feeling the thundering beat beneath my palm.

"You know how to make a girl blush, don't you?"

His fern green eyes pierce my soul and I've all but surrendered myself to him at this point.

"I just say what is on my mind," he says. "Tomorrow night. Can I take you out then?"

"I'd like that very much."

Everett reaches his hand to my cheek, sweeping his thumb from the side of my nose to my ear. The touch of his fingers and the wafting aroma of soap stings me with desire, making me weak in the knees. "Why don't we find your bicycle and put it in the backseat of my car. I'll take you home, or to the corner of your street. Would that be okay?"

Couldn't we just stay here until tomorrow night? I could stare into his eyes for longer than that, but I'd be okay with just a day's time. "Thank you. I would be grateful for the ride."

14

JULY 1941

I COULDN'T BE MORE improper while running down my street, shoes in my hand, hair flying in the wind, and a smile painted along my lips from ear to ear. But Everett's car is in sight. I might become so good at this little game that I'll be able to jump into the car without him having to stop at all.

"You are making me dizzy, doll. What are you doing running all the way down here without shoes on?"

"Well, I'm hiding you from my father, of course. You want to go out tonight, don't you?"

"You know, I don't think you're giving me enough credit. Dads love me. I can turn up the charm," Everett says, flashing me a Hollywood wink while pulling into the nearest driveway to turn around.

"Oh, I'm aware of your ability to be charming, but is it an act, Lieutenant Anderson?"

Everett twists his grip around the steering wheel and leans his head back as if feeling defeat. "What do I have to do to get you to believe me, doll-face? I'm not one of those goons out fishing for broads every night, despite your assumptions."

"My assumptions," I question. "Exactly, what do you think I'm assuming, Lieutenant?" I lift a brow, inquisitively waiting for his response.

I watch the thoughts muster behind his teasing smile. "You

must think I have a reputation that precedes the ones of other celebrities you hear gossip about. You know most of it is rubbish, right?"

I wonder if all stars are trained to deny the stories. I guess I could offer him the benefit of the doubt. "Oh, I know. I just find it surreal that you would want to spend time with me, of all people."

"Just you, beautiful." Everett loops his arm around my neck, pulling me in closer across the front seat.

"Where are we going?"

Everett adjusts his sunglasses as we take a turn toward the setting rays bouncing off the water. "Your favorite place, of course."

"You're taking me to the beach?" I sound giddy at the thought, which is ridiculous seeing as I live on an island.

"Why, where else would you want to go on a beautiful night like tonight?" Every night is beautiful here. It's one thing I've never taken for granted, and one thing I will miss when I choose to leave this island to see more of the world someday.

It's clear Everett puts time into considering my thoughts and feelings, and it's an unfamiliar experience I'm growing fonder of by the day.

The time we have spent together feels like years when it has been just a few occurrences over the last couple of weeks. I've experienced the rush of a schoolgirl crush, wanting what I can't have, and daydreaming about a person who couldn't be more out of my league, but this is different. This chance of a lifetime is staring me in the face and waiting with open arms. My mind tells me I should walk away right after I tell him that this relationship won't end well for either of us, but my heart is hanging on. I believe in living in the current, and I promised myself to think of life as a cluster of last moments—each one being crucial to my happiness and fulfillment. If I listen to my heart, I'll stay right where I am, and even though pain may follow this interlude, I must believe it's worth whatever comes next.

It's hard not to love that Everett already knows my favorite spot, my hiding place. Without hesitation, he pulled up to rocks overlooking the beach. "Don't move a muscle. I am opening your door regardless if you appreciate the gesture, Miss."

A rush of warmth washes through my cheeks as I watch him jog around the front of his car toward my door. He makes me feel like I'm the only other person in the world, and I didn't know anyone could make me feel that way.

"How many hours have you spent sitting on this sand, under this dock, staring at sharp reflections of the moon bouncing off the ocean?" Everett inquires.

"Not enough." It's a simple answer. I could never spend enough time in this spot on the quiet beach. "This place is the gateway between heaven and earth. Where else would I want to be?"

Everett brushes his knuckles against my cheek, then twirls a strand of my hair around his finger. "I have a desire to know every thought spinning around in your busy mind. Listening to the descriptions of life through your eyes is like re-reading a favorite book. I can take comfort knowing your next words will bring a smile to my face and warmth to my heart."

"You have recited many romantic screenplays, haven't you, Lieutenant Anderson?" Maybe he doesn't intend to recall poetic lines from scenes he's read, but I question how anyone could feel so much intensity for me. Plain old me. I'm no different from any other woman. I have accomplished little of anything in my brief life, and I live in fear of my father. These facts are not noble characteristics to fawn over.

Everett doesn't respond with much emotion on his face. He's complacent and seems lost in thought. "Those are my words, Lizzie. It's the way I feel. I don't want you to see me as who I was before I came here. Please. Take me for who I am now—at this moment."

How can I argue when I ask for the same in life? I refuse to discuss the future or the past. Both have unanswered questions that I don't want to think about.

"Of course, I understand. I'm a little scared, I suppose."

Everett stands up from the sand and sweeps the remnants from his pants. "I had no intention of frightening you. What can I do to fix this?"

I stand from the sand too and sweep the back of my dress off as the loose fabric winds around my legs through the wind's pull.

"I'm not afraid of you, Everett. I feel so much, and we've only known each other for such a short time. Of course, without a tomorrow, how will we know what today will bring? I'm scared there's a flaw in my way of thinking."

"A flaw, Miss Lizzie? There isn't a flaw about you, not one I can see. If every day ends up being like today, wouldn't life be magnificent? Imagine never growing old and always feeling this way. Would that make you happy?"

Without a doubt. "Thrilled, indeed."

Everett's fists curl by his side as if panic is rising through him, but as his gaze lowers to my lips, his intent becomes clearer than the glittering sky. I'm left without time to take in a full breath or hold on to the air left in my lungs as he lunges in my direction, curling me into his arms and bringing me flush to his body. His cradling arms lower me as he studies my eyes with intent, as if searching for something he never thought he'd find. The spicy scent of his cologne and mint from his breath heat and cool my skin at the same moment, creating a haze of euphoric comfort. Then, his lips press to mine as our hearts wrestle from within our chests. His hands hold me with what feels like such little effort, yet so much strength. Within his arms, I feel like I could never fall. The wind returns with a push and shove, tangling the fabric of my dress around both pairs of our legs. My hair sweeps across his neck and his hands tighten around my back. I need air, but what's the point? I will gladly embrace a light-headed feeling to allow this moment to continue.

When my feet are flat against the sand and my posture upright, I know the kiss is ending. I want to loop my arms around his neck and hold on a little longer, but I'm a lady and though I choose to think on my own, I must always show a level of grace.

His lips part from mine and the passing breeze leaves my lips stinging with a chill from the loss of his borrowed warmth.

"I'm simply crazy about you, Lizzie."

My hands fold over my chest because I feel breathless just standing in this man's presence. I never imagined feeling this way.

"I'm not sure I can find the proper words to respond." The nerves flickering through my body pull my gaze toward the sand.

"Perhaps, I stole your thoughts," he says.

I glance up through my lashes, catching him biting down on his bottom lip. "My heart, too."

"And to think, we can do this all over again tomorrow as if today never happened."

I want to tell him it will be all I think about until we see each other again. "How will we find each other next time?" I ask.

Everett drops his head and reaches his hand into his pocket, then pulls retrieves a small piece of a note paper with an address scribbled in ink. "You can always find me here before zero nine hundred and after seventeen hundred hours. The side entrance is never used."

I fold the paper into a square and place it into the pocket of my dress. "Well, I won't say I'll see you tomorrow, but if tomorrow is anything like today, then I think we both know what the future holds."

15

OCTOBER 1941

IF LIVING a lie means feeling as though I'm wound up tightly like a spool of thread, day and night with a racing heart, and having the inability to calm the sparks of excitement coursing through my nerves, I suppose there are worse things I could be doing.

The intricate timing of sneaking away and hiding in the shadows from the peepers with big mouths is the only way Everett and I could continue seeing each other throughout the summer. Even after broaching the topic with Dad several times, referencing the idea of dating, not one conversation ended in my favor. I have given up hope of forcing him to understand he's being unreasonable. He's left me no choice but to go about my business in secrecy, at least until I have my nursing certification in hand.

With Everett's barracks in view, I ride around to the back side of the building near the corner stairwell, the one he's always told me to use. Each morning, I remove my heels to hide the clunky sounds of my feet as I jog up the cement stairs. Everett says he never hears me coming, which I sometimes prefer. I find it rather fun to catch him off guard if I show up a few minutes earlier than expected.

However, I suspect he might be on to me as I find him locking his door when I reach the third floor. "Not today, doll-face." I hold my shoes up to my chest, unsure what he means. "I have an idea."

"Well, I can't say I don't love the ideas you come up with." *Spontaneous.* Everett doesn't like routine, which is ironic considering his newfound career path. "What kind of idea takes less than an hour?" This is my last week of classes. Graduation is this weekend, and I'm giddy at the thought of completing three long years of training.

Everett steals the few steps between us and wraps his arm around my waist, pulling me in to kiss me with a soft caress of his lips. His cap slips off his head like it does any time we kiss before work. He's dressed to the nines, and I come along and steal a piece of perfection. "Gosh, you smell nice. You know, plumeria and coconut are my favorite." He retrieves his cap from the ground and dusts off the sides before replacing it on the precise center of his head.

"I know it's your favorite, silly."

Everett places his hand on his heart, closes his eyes and winces in comical pain. "You sure know how to drive a guy wild. I will give you that, Miss Lizzie."

"Well, only you."

I take Everett's hand and tug him toward the stairwell. "Hold on now. I have something I want to give you."

What could he want to give me this early in the morning in the middle of a work week? "You have something for me?" I question.

His smirk tugs to the right like it does when he's being coy or shy, which isn't often. I've only seen the look a few times before. He reaches into the pocket inside his jacket and pulls out a leather-bound book. "I know we're only together for today and we've joked about going steady, but if there ever comes a time when I can't be with you, I want you to have something, so you know I'm thinking about you. Because, even if there isn't a tomorrow, it would take forever for me to forget you." Everett hands me the book. "It's a journal for you to document meaningful moments of your life. Since it's hard to imagine a day without listening to your poetic and worldly thoughts, this book will be like a passage to my soul and you can rest knowing your words will never go unheard."

I can't find the words to speak because I might cry if I open my mouth. I can only wonder if he's preparing to move again and hasn't had the heart to tell me yet. He's afraid something will happen. "This is a wonderful gift," I utter, tracing my fingers along the etched lines of my name he had pressed into the leather. "Is everything okay, Everett? Are you leaving?"

He takes my hand and pulls me into his chest. "I'm not going anywhere right now, but—" Everett's gaze drops to our connected hands.

"But what, Everett?"

He peers back up at me with a look of pain swimming through the murky greens of his eyes. "I'm just so proud of you for completing your nurse training, but I don't want you to think of me as an anchor here. It is what we've always said to one another, right?"

Sure, I said all of that when we first met, but it's been three incredible months. Who knew summer love was something that could happen in real life? The memories we made, in quiet, will stay with me for always.

I haven't mentioned a word about completing my classes because it means I must decide on what comes next, and I only have two options. Either I fly clear across the country to the East Coast or I remain here on base at the hospital where I have spent countless hours for the last three years. I promised myself no one would be a factor in this decision, but my heart aches at the thought of walking away from Everett. Plus, going to the East Coast would require me to leave Dad, James, and Lewis. I don't know if any of us are prepared for that.

"Of course. It means the world to me, knowing you support my dreams, Everett. Honest."

With a small kiss on the cheek, Everett takes my hand and progresses down the open corridor, leading the way. "There's a paratrooper training mission in about fifteen minutes. Do you want to watch?"

"I would love nothing more. I've never seen such a thing." We had little air training on this base until the last couple of months, so while I've seen every other training exercise performed here, I haven't witnessed a man jumping out of a plane.

"This is my dream, you know. I'm going to be a paratrooper if it's the last thing I do."

I hate the thought. Flying planes for the Army is scary enough to think about, never mind jumping out of a perfectly good aircraft. "You may have mentioned this a few times," I say, nudging my shoulder into his arm.

"We can walk, if that's okay with you? It's just a couple of blocks down the road and I'm not sure there will be a good place to park my car."

I stop at the bottom step of his barracks building and slip my shoes on. "Of course."

"It's quite a spectacular sight, you know. I can't wait for you to see this."

I hope I never have to nurse a broken paratrooper back to life. Nurses like to err on the side of caution, but these men—they are always looking for trouble.

* * *

There are soldiers and sailors scattered along the water's edge where we'll be watching a man drop out of a plane. Everett checks his wristwatch and presses up on his toes to search down the shoreline. "Can you see anything?" I ask.

"It looks like the plane is getting ready to take off." I love when Everett lights up with excitement. For someone who has experienced so much luxury in life, he doesn't seem to skip by the insignificant details. He lives to smile, and I might just want to live to see him smile for the rest of my life.

"I hear an engine," I say, trying to see over the rocky barrier between this inlet and the next.

"It's taking off right now," he says, rubbing his hands together.

"Elizabeth Hope Salzberg, I was not expecting to see my daughter at the paratroop testing event this morning."

Dad's voice forces my eyes open wide and my throat to close with apprehension. My head is leaning on Everett's arm. There's no way to cover this up. I twist on my heels to face Dad, afraid to look him in the eyes. "Dad, I—" I should have expected to see him here. I'm the one who doesn't belong.

"Lieutenant Anderson, I've heard so much about you. Of course, none of those wonderful statements had anything to do with you spending time with my daughter."

Everett is going to miss the jump. "Oh, yes, Sir, I've heard many good things about you, as well," Everett says, saluting Dad at attention. I'm not sure how many good things I've shared about Dad other than the issues that shadow over everything else.

"Elizabeth, may I have a word with you please?"

"Dad, I'm sure this can wait just a few moments for us to all see what we came here for, couldn't it?" Dad stretches his neck as if needing air between his skin and the inside of his collar, then clears his throat. He's staring at me with so much anger, and the hurt in his eyes makes little sense to me. I'm a grown woman. He's forced me to hide my life from him. I wish he could see what he's done and understand why I am the way I am. This isn't an act of rebellion; I'm living my life because it's mine to live.

It's hard to hold my focus on the man jumping from the plane. I'm glad to see Everett is enjoying the display, but I know we're both minutes from an interrogation for ridiculous reasons and I would do anything to prevent Everett from having to endure what's next.

The crowd of soldiers and sailors are cheering at the sight of a parachute which I feel could have opened a couple seconds sooner, but I have other things to worry about right now.

"Elizabeth, a word," Dad repeats.

"I'll be right back," I whisper to Everett.

I follow Dad several feet away from where we were standing, to a quiet area where no one else will hear our conversation. "What in the world is going through your head? Have you lost your mind?"

"No, Dad, I've lost the desire to argue my rights with you. I'm not a child. I'm a grown woman about to embark on a career that will allow me to care for others the way Mom did. It shouldn't be your decision of who I choose to spend my time with."

Dad straightens his shoulders, and his neck stiffens. "How dare you speak to me this way? When you live on your own, you can do as you please, but while I still financially support you, I believe I'm entitled to some say in the foolish decisions you make."

"Foolish?" I'm doing my best to keep the volume of my voice low. I know how this could end if anyone were to hear our conversation. "I love him, Dad. We've been going steady for almost three months and I haven't been able to share that with you because you would rather keep me locked up in our house like a wife without a husband and a mother without children. It's my turn to live, and it isn't fair for you to hold me back."

"You don't know who you're getting involved with, Elizabeth. He isn't just another soldier here on base. That boy—"

"He's a man—a good man, one you know little about, and aside from that fact, you never let me date anyone on the base. That was unfair too."

"Elizabeth, I'm furious over your secrets and lies. I have done nothing but try my hardest to give you the best life possible and this is the thanks I get."

My life felt perfect until Mom died. Dad's soul died with her, and nothing has come close to that consoling feeling since. We move through life in a spell of breaths and few words. It isn't something I consider a good life.

"Dad, I received a job offer in Boston," I say. I didn't plan to tell him this information until after receiving my certification this weekend, but I suppose the news doesn't matter much. "And, well —I'm thinking about taking it."

It's one thing to prevent me from going steady with a man on base, but it's another to interfere with my career. It's something he wouldn't do unless I was enlisting in the military. His only wish is for me to have a civilian career as a nurse. I'm guessing Everett doesn't sound like the worst idea to him right now.

CURRENT DAY - OCTOBER 2018

THE JOURNAL—I thought Makena gave it to me. I lean toward my nightstand and gather the soft leather-bound book in my hand. A desire to hold it up to my nose reminds me of a time when I used to inhale the sweet scent of leather when there wasn't any other aroma worth inhaling.

I trace my finger down each embossed letter of my name, recalling the look in Everett's eyes when he handed me the empty pages to fill out all those years ago. I could have been a writer and a nurse. He made it so I could have it all.

DECEMBER 1941

WEEKS OF SILENCE followed the inevitable rendezvous and my completion of nursing school. There wasn't a celebration or a sense of accomplishment.

Life has continued to push forward, leaving me with nothing but an angry parent and a life-altering decision I must make between the Atlantic and Pacific coast—staying here in an unapproved relationship with Everett or leaving him behind for a career opportunity I should feel grateful to have.

I knew it was only a matter of time before Dad would catch onto me about Everett. I just didn't know when or how long we might have to enjoy each other's company without stress.

After the mortifying scene at the paratrooper exhibition, so many thoughts came to mind. I had a lot to fight for, but with the one person I would never want to fight. Dad and I argued for days. I eventually told him that if he felt the need to kick me out because of my differing beliefs on dating, going steady, or Everett in general, I would leave without a fight. He knows I don't have many options for places to stay, but he is also aware I wouldn't have too much trouble finding someone to take me in, and the small talk around base would be worse than the current situation we're living.

Our conversations are brief within the house; nothing more than: hello, goodbye, goodnight, and thank you. He stopped asking where I was going when I left, and I lost interest in hiding my comings and goings. Everett seems determined to have a man-to-man talk with Dad, but I've requested that he doesn't engage in this nonsense. If Dad didn't make such a deal out of a relationship, Everett could join us for dinner at night and get to know the people I love most, but instead, the boys and I often have secret family dinners at diners without Dad. James and Lewis are fond of Everett, and their feelings toward him mean the world to me. They have both attempted to talk Dad down from his irrational thoughts but have gotten nowhere. I accept that Dad may never approve of anyone for me, and it will drive a wedge between us that we won't be able to repair.

"There she is," Everett says, greeting me with open arms. It's unusual to find him out of uniform, but it's Saturday night, and we're going to see a picture at the theatre. Even when not dressed for work, he looks like a heartthrob who has fallen off a movie set. With his taupe fitted dress trousers, a matching vest and bow tie embellished by the vibrant white glow of his button-down shirt, he is sensational and will surely be a sight for sore eyes tonight among the ladies downtown. Everett doesn't give me reason to worry about the others who noticed his presence here. The tight grip of his hand around mine is all I ever need to feel like nothing could ever go wrong. Together, we walk on water, and though it's not always practical, the sparks between us make me forget about everything else. Love can do such crazy things.

He's leaning against the passenger side door of his car, waiting for me to fall into his embrace. "Sorry for making you wait an extra minute. I was waiting on the silly kitchen timer so I could take their casserole out of the oven. I thought I had it all timed out to perfection, but —"

Everett wraps his arms around me and kisses my forehead. "Don't be ridiculous. I've heard some women make a man wait for hours on her while she powders her face to go out for an evening."

"Oh, no, I could never spend that much time preparing to go out so that I can come home and wash it all away."

I straighten my posture to step back along the sidewalk so

Everett can open the car door. "How is your father this evening?" Everett asks as he does whenever he picks me up at the house.

"I'm not sure. He's had his head buried in work all day. I poked my head in to say goodbye and let him know dinner was on the table."

I pinch my skirt to slide into the car, but before Everett can close the door, Dad steps outside onto the front step. He hasn't been so forward since the exhibition, and I'm terrified of what he is about to say. "Are you truly going to the theatre tonight?" Dad calls out.

Everett clicks his heels together as if it's an automated response and salutes Dad. The gesture makes me want to roll my eyes, but I refrain. "Yes, sir, I will have her home before ten. Is that all right, Sir?"

Dad slips his hands into his pockets and rolls back on his heels. "Maybe you would like to stay and join us for dinner instead?" I'm questioning if I'm hearing Dad correctly because those words would never form on his lips.

"Dad, we have plans with friends tonight."

"We could postpone," Everett whispers to me.

"No," I reply in a harsh breath.

"He's trying to make amends, Lizzie. Let's take the chance."

Everett did something I never imagined he would do. "Sir, we would love to join you for supper tonight. Lizzie was just saying how wonderful the casserole came out."

"Why, I never!" My exasperation is uncontrollable in response to this uncomfortable "peace offering."

"Something seems awry with your father. I'll make it up to you. I promise, doll-face." It's hard to say no to his big green eyes when they're staring at me like that, but he can clearly see how furious I am that he jumped at my father's first invitation. It's the least he deserves now—the very least. The only thing that's off about Dad is the rude plan he probably has up his sleeve to trap Everett and threaten him to stay away from me.

"Just wonderful," I mumble, swiveling out of the car. "Tomorrow morning, we'll go up to Puu Ualakaa Lookout to have breakfast at sunrise like we've been discussing. How does that sound?"

It sounds like an enchanting distraction from this infuriating moment, but we have been talking about a sunrise picnic for weeks now, and I would love the opportunity with him. I all but groan before responding with cordiality. "All right, Mr. Hollywood. You win this time, but next time —"

"I can never win more than I've already won, gorgeous," he says, reaching out to take my hand. He's unashamed to walk into my house, claiming me as his even with my father inside.

Once inside, Dad pulls out the two extra chairs at the table. "Your brothers won't be home in time for dinner. They had a drill to tend to." I suppose this could be the reason Dad wanted us to eat with him. No one wants to dine alone. I can't blame him, I guess, but he made his bed in this situation.

"A drill?" Everett asks, removing his cap while brushing the soil from his shoes on the entryway mat.

"Yes," Dad responds.

Everett and Dad exchange a look I can't decipher and one I don't care to see. "Is everything okay?" I ask.

"Of course," Dad says without skipping a beat. His eyes tell a different story, one he doesn't think I can interpret, but there's something on his mind, and he's nervous about whatever it might be.

Everett doesn't appear to be the slightest bit nervous, and yet I feel the need to go powder my nose because of the perspiration creeping up my neck. With a deep inhale through my nose and a slow exhale out my mouth, I do what I can to calm myself. I go to the cabinets to gather enough plates for the three of us, but as I place the china down onto the table, Dad stands up. "Elizabeth, sit down. I'll take care of the rest."

"I'm happy to help, Sir," Everett offers.

"No, no, I'm all set. Thank you, son."

Son. I smell a rat.

It doesn't take long before we're all sitting across from one another at the table, preparing to take our first bites. "How are things going here for you on this base, Lieutenant Anderson? I've heard nothing but wonderful feedback on the Army Air Corps program so far. It seems you men have everything in great working order."

Small talk. Is that what this is? A way to waste time while we
eat our meals so Dad can speed up to the part of the night where
he sends Everett home. "The men in my squadron are super. We
all get along just fine and have made a lot of progress with
training over the last few months."

"Good, good, I'm glad to hear it." Dad takes a few bites of the
casserole, and Everett follows his every move as inferior rank will
do no matter the situation. "It's a relief to know this base is
becoming well rounded with expertise and support. Are you
enjoying Oahu so far?"

This chatter is the most I've heard Dad speak in weeks, and I
wish I could figure out the meaning behind this ploy.

"Oh yes, I'm very fond of the island. It's much different
from the last couple of places I trained. The scenery is
unsurpassable here." Everett throws me a spry glance and wink
as Dad peers down to scoop up another bite. This charmer
doesn't miss an opportunity to make me blush. It's as if he has a
goal count set for the day. After spending months with Everett,
my feelings, desire, and yearning to be with him has only
grown.

"It is a wonderful place to live, isn't it, Elizabeth?" Ah, Dad's
intention is crystal clear. This unexpected supper is his
opportunity to discuss the decision I have less than a week to
make. The hospital in Boston and the hospital here offered me a
position to join their staff after the new year which is a month
from now. However, I owe my decision to the chosen hospital
three weeks before a start date.

"Of course," I reply, taking my turn to fill my mouth with
food.

"There aren't many places in the United States where you find
perfect year-round temperatures. In fact, I'm not sure I could
settle down elsewhere after living here for so long. To imagine a
life where the beach is more than a few minutes away or the
temperatures fall below thirty degrees, I often wonder how people
live in those conditions."

The temptation to clear my throat in response to the amount
of bologna coming from Dad's mouth is astounding. We have
gone on vacations to see snow-covered mountain-tops, and he

hates the beach. In fact, he would be much happier if I never went to the beach here at all, and I don't have a clue why that is.

"Oh, it's not all that bad, Sir. Every part of this country has its pros and cons, I suppose. Though I might agree that Hawaii is hard to compete with in terms of perfect weather and scenery."

"Precisely," Dad says.

"Imagine wanting to move to New England in the dead of winter. Only a fool would be—"

"Enough," I snap, tossing my napkin down onto the table. "How dare you prompt an agenda using supper as a cover-up for your selfish reasons? We had plans with friends tonight, and you persuaded us to stay here so you wouldn't have to eat alone. I can only imagine you must have told Lewis and James not to come home for a bit so you could take this time to make your move."

"Elizabeth, pardon me, but I don't think it's necessary to be acting so irrational in front of our guest right now. Please, take your seat."

"You cannot tell me what to do any longer, Dad. I am a grown woman and don't deserve that type of treatment." The discomfort displaying within Everett's wide stare is a blatant plea for me to pause this conversation until a later point, but the words are flowing like a waterfall, and I'm not sure I can contain my anger any longer. "My decision concerning which position I will accept has no bearing on the weather or location. I will receive unique experiences in each hospital, and those are the facts I am focusing on."

For the first time since I have been offered the positions, I notice an inflection of disdain glistening within Everett's eyes. We have had conversations about what is best for each of us versus what would be wonderful for the two of us together. The decision has been impossible to make. I don't want to leave Everett, nor my family, despite Dad's behavior at the moment, but Boston would open up a new world of possibilities, new adventures, sights, and the reputation of those hospitals cannot be beat. Some might call me a fool for choosing any other place to begin my career.

"It's not safe out on the East Coast right now, Elizabeth. I don't know how else to make you understand. You act as though you live in a safe bubble here on this island because soldiers, sailors, and airmen surround you. What you don't realize is what is awaiting outside of this island. You are a Jewish woman walking around in a world that sees us as the enemy. Anti-Semitism may not be as obvious here in the United States, but I promise you, even though the thoughts are quiet, they are present more than you can imagine."

I place my palms down on the table, the friction causes a hollow thud louder than intended. "How is it that anti-Semitism is obvious to you but no one else? What do you know that I don't?" I question, trying my best to keep my tone down.

"You heard what Lindbergh said just a few months ago. Maybe you aren't aware of the uprising caused by his blame against the Jewish people for this war, but it exists in places you can't see unless you are there. And I don't want you there."

I shake my head with utter disappointment. "There was a brawl in New York. It's over. I can't live in fear of an occurrence that has come and gone. It's not fair to ask that of me and you know it."

"Elizabeth, they were Nazi supporters. Aside from that, there is no one for you to go to if you find trouble on the East Coast. In another situation, at a different time, I would encourage you to spread your wings and fly, but I've already lost one love of my life, and I refuse to lose another. My job on earth is to keep you safe, and it is not safe outside of this base right now, despite what you assume."

My heart pounds so hard, every bone in my body aches. This career path was supposed to be my decision, no one else's.

"Sir, is something going on that we are unaware of?" Everett inquires.

Dad's gaze falls to his half-empty plate of food. "No, we don't know what tomorrow might bring. That's all." He isn't looking Everett in the eyes. Dad doesn't speak without making direct eye-contact. Not unless he's lying.

"Elizabeth says the same, but with all due respect, Sir, if we don't know what tomorrow might bring, why should we live in fear of the unknown?"

Dad's face burns with a red hue, a distinct emotion I don't

recall seeing before. He drops his fork to the glass plate and the shattering clink echoes within the dangling crystals of the chandelier above our heads. He presses the napkin against his mouth and tosses it onto his plate. "Because I said so, dammit, that's why." With his final statements on the matter, Dad stands and retreats to his bedroom, then slams the door with unnecessary force.

"I think there might be something going on here," Everett whispers.

I slap my hands down against my lap, frustrated beyond words. "Why, what do you mean?"

Everett folds his hands, resting them on the table as if to display a sense of calm while I'm foaming at the mouth. "I'm not sure, but I'll see what I can do about finding out."

Dad got his way. He spoiled the night for us all. "We will need to postpone our breakfast plans for tomorrow morning now, I assume?" It's hard to force a sense of cheer after such a mortifying scene, but I feel like all my opportunities of joy become stolen in some way or another.

Everett places his hand on top of mine. "No, of course not. I wouldn't miss the opportunity for anything in the world, gorgeous. Meet me outside at zero six hundred hours tomorrow morning, and we'll go."

His agreement to keep our plans almost helps me forget about the fit we just witnessed, but I doubt my mind will rest easy tonight while stewing on each word Dad said. "I'm looking forward to the morning, then."

I pause for a moment, preparing to clear the plates, but an unsettling shadow falls over my shoulders, weighing me down to the seat. "Everett, is there any truth to what he said?" I turn to face him, needing to see the answer within his eyes.

He lifts my hand and holds it between his, offering me warmth and comfort, a gesture to ease the blow of whatever he has to say next. "I'm not exactly sure, Lizzie. A lot is going on in the world right now, and it's hard to assume the safety of anyone's location. You know I'm not the one who will hold you back from fulfilling your desires, but if the question is about safety, I can't say I disagree with your father."

"So, you agree with him then?"

Everett lifts my knuckles to his lips. I assume he is trying to ease the anger he must see rising through my burning cheeks. "Don't ask me to take sides, please, darling."

It pains me to pull my hand from this, but this isn't fair. "I didn't, but it's clear whose side you have chosen." I take my hand from Everett's, placing it down on my lap. "Well, then I guess it's settled."

Everett leans forward and presses his finger below my chin. "Look at me, doll," he says with a look full of empathy. "I will support whatever decision you make. I might worry like crazy about you, but this is your life and your right to decide. I want to know you're safe. I wouldn't forgive myself if I didn't express my concerns, and something happened to you. I'm sure you must understand where I'm coming from?"

"Are you saying this because I'm a Jewish woman or because I'm a woman who wants to move across the country to fulfill a career I am passionate about?"

"I won't lie to you, Lizzie, both reasons should be considered when you make this decision."

I feel empty inside, like someone has flipped me upside down and is shaking me to pieces. Mom wouldn't give in to fear. She would stand tall and ferociously show her pride to be a Jewish woman. How can I take a step back and undo what she spent her life working toward? Why does it matter who I am? "This world is despicable. No one can be who they are or want to be without criticism or law standing in the way. We are to be what the world dictates, and I'm done succumbing to conformity."

18

DECEMBER 1941

THE SONGBIRDS outside my window are reviving me from the few hours of sleep I stole after spending most of the night tossing and turning as I stirred over the commotion at the dinner table. I'm not sure if what I'm feeling is anger, resentment, or suppression. I suppose it could be all three. I must wonder if any of us have choices in life, or are we just led to believe we do?

The arguments between Dad and me aren't new, but Everett's opinion took me by surprise. It was challenging to say goodnight to him because I was at a loss for words, which doesn't happen often.

Part of me wonders if Everett was taking Dad's side to appear as a figure of authority, or maybe he felt the need to prove his worth as the man in my life, protecting me at all costs. But after Dad left the room, Everett and I spoke in private. That moment, realizing his opinion hadn't changed, made it hard to assume anything more than the fact of him agreeing with Dad.

Of course, I could very well be wrong, but it's a tough concept to digest when I feel I should be independent and enjoy the liberty of choosing the path I want to follow. *Freedom.*

Maybe someone should search the word's definition in a dictionary because the meaning seems to have become lost or forgotten.

I'm going to have bags under my eyes today. I should ring Everett and tell him I'm feeling ill. The thought of breaking our plans yanks at my heart. Even though I'm distraught about the conversation we had last night, I still want to see him and spend the morning together. This must be how a woman falls under the hypnotic control of a man. She falls in love and becomes too weak to do anything more than smile and agree to his every whim.

The decision is mine to make.

I blink at the time on my clock, telling myself I have less than a half-hour to get myself ready before Everett pulls up out front to wait for me. A cold splash of water against my face might help get me moving.

One by one, I unwind the curlers from my hair, realizing I twisted them tighter than usual last night—a side-effect of going to bed frustrated and angry. With one glance in the mirror, I realize I look like the childhood version of Shirley Temple with her tight barrel curls and dimpled cheeks. I run my brush through each tendril, yanking at each spiral. With a mess of locks to deal with, I haven't had a chance to paint a coat of mascara over my lashes when I see the glow of headlights outside my window.

As usual, Everett is right on time, never a minute early or late. I take my lipstick and smooth it over my lips, check my teeth for remnants of pigment, slip on a sweater, and grab my purse and shoes to sneak out of the house before Dad notices my footsteps.

I tiptoe through the cool dew-covered grass, inhaling the lush aroma of damp plumerias, as I make my way closer to Everett's car. I spot him standing by the passenger door with eager eyes and a radiant smile. He always finds a way to make my heart melt, even in my fit of exasperation. "Aloha. Good morning," I whisper.

"Aloha, doll-face," he greets me. "Gosh, who needs the sun when I have a pretty little thing like you to light up the day? The Burgundy of your sweater makes your eyes light up." There he goes again, saying things I can't move passed. He presses his lips to my cheek before inviting me into his car. "I missed you."

I want to tell him I slept poorly because last night upset me so much, but I bite my tongue for the moment. He closes the door and rushes around to his side, smoothly closing himself inside. "I missed you too." My response feels delayed, but I always miss him when we're not together despite my frustration.

While placing his hands on the steering wheel, Everett pulls in a sharp breath through his nose, hinting at a sign of anguish. "I know you're upset about what I said last night. Am I right?"

To think that there is a type of man who can read a woman's mind ... well, he must be wise beyond his years. I sigh and drop my gaze to my interwoven gloved fingers. "Well, yes, I'm still quite bothered over the conversation that took place." There's no reason to lie about the way I feel. I always thought Mom should have been more honest with Dad about how she felt about specific topics.

Everett twists his head toward me and takes one of my hands into his. "Lizzie, I shouldn't have interfered. I love you, that's all."

"Well, I appreciate your words. Thank you for understanding," I reply, trying to sound proper and cordial in favor of my argument.

"But to be fair, it is slightly your fault."

"Well, I'll be. How in the world do you suppose that?" I argue.

"It's entirely your fault that you made me fall in love with you. You took away my control to be a man of restraint. Some might even say you stole my freedom of choosing whether I fall in love with a beautiful, smart, sassy, outspoken woman like yourself, but what's the point in arguing. I allowed it to happen, right?"

His words permeate my tired mind. I believe he's trying to explain that he allowed my influence to take over. I wouldn't have thought I could have such an effect on someone.

"I see." I try to stifle the smile growing across my lips.

"If I didn't want to fall in love with you, I could have walked away."

"You mean to say you could have avoided heartbreak," I remind him.

"Spending these months with you is well worth any form of heartbreak I might experience beyond today." Everett veers away from the curb, cruising in near silence toward the end of the street.

I twist my body to stare at the profile of his face; a silhouette within the darkness. "How do you always know just the right words to make me forget what I was angry about?"

He peers over at me for a brief second. "The last thing I want to do is upset you, but I promised you I would be honest no matter what. Honesty is our foundation, isn't it?"

The truth should be something I appreciate, respect, and consider—but not allow it to dictate my decision. "You're a smart man, Everett."

"I wouldn't go that far, but my respect for you goes beyond what I can express. I just want you to know what I'm thinking. You're a resilient woman, and I know you can handle more than most might give you credit for, which means I don't doubt you will make the best decision for yourself. In fact, I find this trait to be one of your finest qualities."

As hard as it is to admit I may have been wrong, I should have respected his feelings last night and took his words for what they were—his opinion. His thoughts mean more to me than I might have guessed.

"I appreciate your honesty. Your explanation didn't come as a surprise. Nothing you said was foreign or something I hadn't considered because I'm fighting a battle that will make me a stronger person. But trying to balance my desires with safety feels impossible some days. My mother wanted me to be a powerful woman, independent, free of other's rules. Now, I must decide what that means for me."

"I respect that, and I would never stand in the way of your decision. I hope you understand this," he says.

By the time we're pulling into the lookout point's parking area, I'm feeling relief from the aggravation that tore me apart all night. "I haven't been here in so long, since I was a kid maybe," I tell Everett.

"Well, I've never been here at all, so I'm looking forward to the view you've been describing. I packed us breakfast."

I almost forgot about breakfast and hadn't considered who would bring the food. I should have offered, but the thought never crossed my mind. "You did?"

"Yes, Ma'am, I got up a little early and made some pancakes

and eggs that are hopefully still warm. I also have a thermos full of coffee, so we have all the important elements for a perfect breakfast with a beautiful view."

"You cooked?"

"As far as I know," he says with a grin. "To be fair, I usually only cook for myself, but I haven't complained much recently. Plus, I believe a man should know how to cook, shouldn't he?"

I can't contain my laughter, even if it pokes at my heart to imagine him eating alone.

"Well, of course. I just don't know many men who will do much of anything in the kitchen, including cooking an egg. So, I'm pleasantly surprised by your gesture." We've been together for almost five months, and the conversation about cooking hasn't come up once. I assumed he was much like James, Lewis, and Dad when tending to domestic chores. We've always gone to the mess hall or out to a restaurant. I've cooked for him occasionally, but I insisted each of those times.

Everett makes his way over to my car door and offers me a hand before reaching into the back seat for a picnic basket and blanket I hadn't noticed.

"This is very thoughtful and sweet."

We don't have to walk far to find the perfect spot to watch the sunrise over the ocean. Everett places the picnic basket down and smooths out the blanket for us to sit on. I reach for the basket, but he pulls it away, insisting on serving the items. "I'm quite capable, Miss Lizzie."

He places two plates on the blanket, then a tin, and a couple of jars filled with the food he cooked up. "This looks delicious, Everett." The tins are still warm to the touch, and the coffee is steaming when he pours it into two mugs.

A flare of sunlight peeks over the horizon in a flat glowing orange line. It's blinding against the fading darkness. "Do you ever experience moments you want to make sure to remember and carry with you forever?" I ask.

Everett takes a small sip of his coffee and grins. "There have been so many of them lately. I can only hope they all stick with me."

"Aside from these last several months, I've only had a handful of memories I've wanted to keep. This habit I have may sound silly, but when there is something remarkable happening, I like to imagine painting the scene in my mind; noting every detail, even down to the number of leaves there are on a flower's stem or how the hues from a melting sun change and morph into different shades just before the sky turns black."

"That's a wonderful way to remember a moment," he says.

I lose myself in thought, trying to recall the last time I painted a memory before meeting Everett. It isn't hard to remember, though. "Her hand was cold, not quite like ice, but like she needed a pair of gloves. Her fingers were weak, and the beds of her nails were a pale blue mixed with a hint of purple. I'm not sure if her nails always looked that way because she was vigilant about keeping her nails painted with bright red polish. I stroked my thumb along her knuckles, hoping I was relieving at least some of her pain." She seemed to relax when I tried to soothe her. I didn't know what else to do. "I pressed her hand against my cheek, feeling the silky soft skin that wiped away so many of my tears in the past. I needed her to wipe my tears away at that moment, but she was too weak. Her hand smelled faintly of soap and the creme I had massaged onto her skin the night before. She struggled to open her eyes wide enough to look at me, but the amber coloring of her irises against the ghostly color of her pale skin was still as vibrant as it was when she was healthy."

"Those details — I can picture her, Lizzie," Everett says.

"She wouldn't have wanted you to see her looking that way," I choke up a quiet chuckle. "I had never seen Mom without makeup before that time, but she was a natural beauty, even without the pigment of blood pumping through her skin the way it should have been. I needed to know I would not forget the way she looked. I needed to know that whenever I would close my eyes for the rest of my life, I would have the clearest image of her, even if it was the way she appeared in those last days. Her soul was still living inside of her, exhaling the life I wanted to hold on to. I would stare at each freckle on her face, each line left behind from stress, the few eyelashes that didn't curl like the others, and the deep shade of pink of her earlobes from the heavy earrings she often wore. Her lips were pale compared to what I usually saw, but the shape of her cupid's bow was the same. She already looked like an angel."

Everett is staring into my eyes, or maybe through my eyes, as if he's lost. My words might have reminded him of his mother, I suppose. "Despite makeup or sickness, it sounds like you look exactly like her down to those few eyelashes that curl differently than the others." He smiles and takes my hand. "You must promise to always keep memories like that. If we're ever to be apart, I'll know I can relive the moments with you when we're back together."

"What about the times I'm with you—the ones I paint pictures of to keep locked away in my mind forever?"

"I'll want the reminders of those too. You can keep them in the journal. They'll be safe there."

"Absolutely. Perhaps I should start the first page with this moment; it's a beautiful portrait in my mind."

"How do you do it? How do you see every fine detail? Teach me, Lizzie."

I shrug because I'm not sure how it happens; how every detail of everything around me forms into a movie in my mind, but it does and locked there, in a frozen moment.

"I notate aromas, the temperature, sensations of anything touching my skin, the taste on my tongue, the sounds of what is nearby and what is far off in the distance, and the color pallet of the surrounding landscape. I don't know. It's the same as when I write. I close my eyes, and I can recall all the little details. There is so much to experience in life, and I'm afraid of missing out on the slightest detail."

"That's an incredible talent," he says, his eyes glossy as if mesmerized by my explanation.

"Try it. I'm sure you're quite capable of the same."

"Oh, I don't know."

"Close your eyes," I say, running my hand down the side of his cheek. "What do you smell?"

He takes a moment to collect his thoughts before speaking. "I smell vanilla, coffee beans, a variety of botanicals, and the sea mist. I didn't know the sea mist had a smell, but it's salty, I suppose."

"And what do you taste?" I ask through a whisper.

He's quicker to answer this time. "I taste the flavors of coffee and syrup from the pancakes." With slow blinks, Everett's eyes soften, admiring me as if he's trying to memorize my features but leans in and claims my lips. His tongue meets mine, and my heart races with desire as he cups his hands around my cheeks. "You," he mutters against my mouth. "I taste you."

It's hard to consider any other sensation when feeling like this, and I'll happily forget about the sounds and colors of the world if I can remember this—the touch of his lips, his tongue, the sweet taste of sugar. The moment lasts for what seems like minutes, but he pulls away quicker than I wanted and darts his gaze out toward the ocean. "Is everything okay?" I ask.

"Shh," he hushes me, holding his finger up to his mouth. "Do you hear that?"

I close my eyes to focus on whatever sound he's hearing, but I can't discern much other than a low rumble of wind in the distance. "It's just the breeze because we're up high."

"No," he says, staring with intensity toward the horizon. "No, no, that sound is not from the wind."

"What do you mean?" I ask, trying to laugh away the nerves from his apparent apprehension.

Everett stands up from the blanket and holds his hand over his eyes to shield the abundance of light leaking over the horizon, but we can't see much since a cluster of clouds are hovering over the water. He lowers his hand in a slow movement. "Lizzie, get into the car."

"Why? What's going on?"

"Get in the car right now. Go."

I lean down to stack the plates back into the picnic basket. "I'll just clean this up," I say.

"No, leave it there. Let's go."

"Everett, we can't just leave this—"

He takes my wrist within his hand and pulls me away from where we were sitting. "I'm sorry. Just, please listen."

"I don't understand."

He opens my car door and helps me inside faster than I would typically move. Everett is in his seat within seconds, burning rubber as we back out of the parking spot. My mind is racing with questions he won't answer, and I'm still unsure of what he heard.

"I don't understand either, but I need to find out," he says.

19

DECEMBER 1941

THE ROADS ARE blurry as we take sharp turns down every side street. Everett's eyes fixate on the sky more than the road in front of us. My heart is racing so hard. I feel like I've been running through the thick morning fog. My knuckles ache against my grip of the door handle, and I'm staring toward the horizon, waiting for answers—ones I'm fearful to know. In the time Everett and I have known each other, I have never seen his complexion so pale, his eyes this wide and unblinking, nor his breaths so erratic. We were a few miles away from reaching the entrance of the base, but we made it from the lookout point to the gate within seven minutes.

The moment Everett finds a location to pull over, a blaring alarm encircles us, stealing our breath as we look toward the sky for more answers. As the siren continues, we receive our answer:

AIR RAID ON PEARL HARBOR.
THIS IS NOT A DRILL.

Dad, James, and Lewis—I don't know where they are.

An air raid—it's part of military training. The civilians are often sitting in the dark, waiting for information. There's protocol.

There's meaning, but I know none of what to expect, what is to come, how bad this might be.

Everett tugs my hand, pulling me across the front seat of his car until we're both standing firmly on the dirt-ledge overlooking the water for more visibility.

The low rumble that terrorized Everett was many more miles away than we were from the base. Even with the car's engine running, the rumble is amplifying and growing into an eruption. The earth is quaking from the sky, and the shuddering movements, accompanied by piercing whistles and baritone thumps, vibrate through every limb of my body.

The instant I spot a cluster of low-flying aircraft gliding along the horizon, I shout with every ounce of strength I have. "Everett, are those warplanes?" My question feels so innocent compared to the bewilderment fleeting through his wildly flashing eyes.

"Yes, they are," Everett shouts, taking my hand within his. "I'm not sure what they're doing, or who these people are, flying over Pearl like this."

I've never seen a foreign plane hovering so low over the water before. As if the distance between the horizon and the spot we're standing is only a hundred yards, the planes gain speed and skim the low bearing clouds above us.

"Everett—" I try to point at the symbol below the planes' wings, but I must cover my eyes from the debris whipping around us.

"Japanese aircraft," he shouts.

The red sun, the vivid blood-red matching circles beneath each wing mark their presence without a doubt. The squeal and whine stab like knives into my ears as I struggle to glance up at Everett, waiting for a reaction, information, or a plan because I don't understand what's happening.

"What should we do?" I yell, but I'm sure Everett cannot hear my voice over the roar.

Everett closes his eyes, grabs my hand, and he mumbles through the words:

"Hail Mary, full of Grace, the Lord is with thee ..."

He's praying. I believe he's begging for our mercy.

For mercy, from whatever is about to happen.

Dad spent nights praying for Mom to pull through toward the end of her illness. I can recall the words:

"She-ma Yisrael, Adonai eloheinu, Adonai echad;
    Hear Israel, the Lord is our God, the Lord is
    One"—a plea for protection. It didn't work
    then. Please, God, help us now.

Smoke rises and falls from every direction as the earth shatters beneath our feet, tossing us to our knees. Everett lunges on top of me, pulling me into a ditch beneath the flat surface of land. His body is covering mine, and it's hard to breathe. I want to cry and scream out, but for what? He's helping me in the only way he can, by shielding my body ... "Everett," I groan through the muffled weight.

"Lizzie, I have to get you out of here," he shouts.

He pulls me from the ditch, holding his arms around me so tightly, I'm unable to panic as much as I feel the need. "What's happening?" I cry out.

"We're under—"

I can't hear a thing over the roaring shrills above.

Everett tugs me toward the car, and I push myself to move quicker, so he doesn't have to worry about me lagging. "I'm bringing you home, Lizzie. You need to find a safe place. Do you understand?" His shouts are thunderous, but I can only see his lips moving, and the horror reeling through his eyes. His words float in the wind on ear-piercing bursts of sound.

"No, Everett. No! I'm not going home. I need to help. Take me with you."

"The entire air base is under attack, Lizzie. I'm not bringing you down there."

"My father and brothers are probably heading to the shipyard now if they aren't already there. What if they were hit? I cannot go home, Everett. Do not bring me there," I demand.

Everett slams his palms against the steering wheel as sweat

trickles down between the swollen veins of his neck. "Elizabeth," he grits out.

"Don't say it, Everett. Don't."

"You need to understand, I love you, and if anything happens, I won't—I don't know what to do."

"I will not sit at home while our base is under attack, Everett. I'm a trained medical professional, and I need to help. You must listen. I love you, too, but neither of us is safe no matter where we go or what we do."

Everett doesn't continue arguing, and I can tell by the direction he's driving, he's no longer heading to my house. The sirens grow louder along with the shattering metallic pings shooting through my nerves. The destruction isn't ending, and the attack is growing louder and larger by the second. Though it feels like hours have gone by since we spotted the first plane, it's hardly been fifteen minutes as we pull into the Naval shipyard.

We dash out of the car from our respective sides, meeting in front, watching the surreal scene playing out before us. People are running—running for their lives. Soldiers, Sailors, and Nurses are scattering in every direction as if blindfolded.

I don't know whether to run and hide or join the force of help. Panic is consuming my body. By instinct, I believe I should find safety, but with a sense of defiance in my genes, and strength will not allow me to sit back and watch.

The smoke-filled sky appears freckled with a flock of swarming birds.

Those are not birds flying in astonishing synchronizing patterns, though.

They are warplanes intending to destroy everything around us.

From the corner of my eye, I spot makeshift tents popping up. I don't know if those tents will be safe from the hawks above, but every second we stand here, the smoke becomes more profuse, encircling us from every direction. "I must help them," I scream out to Everett. I turn on my heels in search of the best path to move.

"Lizzie," Everett bellows.

"I need to go help those nurses," I reply.

"Lizzie," he hollers again, grabbing my elbow and spinning me around. His hands press against my cheeks and his eyebrows knit together. "This is bad. This is terrible, sweetheart." His words are only words. The fear is clear within his beautiful eyes. We may die trying to help or die trying to hide. He knows this to be the truth. "I want to protect you."

"You need to protect yourself, Everett, never mind the both of us. Look around. People need us more than we need each other right now."

Everett's hands tighten around my cheeks. His gaze darts toward every thud and zing, but for a quick second, he casts his stare into my eyes as if sharing his soul—giving me every part of him. "If I lose you, Elizabeth, please know that the time I've spent with you has been worth every second I've been alive on this earth." I try to shake my head, wishing he wouldn't be speaking this way. We need hope. "Listen, baby, if today is my last, I need to thank you for being my yesterday. You are my world, my one and only, and if the worst finds me, I am one lucky son-of-a-gun to die having felt the way I do about you."

I slap my hands against his chest. "Don't you dare say goodbye to me. Don't you dare, Everett Anderson. This isn't it— this isn't how our story ends. It's just the part where we prove what we're worth to this world. Let's do what we were both trained to do and fight for our people. You will have me tomorrow, Everett. There will be a tomorrow." I'm clenching his shirt into my fists, wishing to believe every word that is spilling from my numb lips.

"Tell me you believe me. Say it."

Everett closes his eyes and presses his forehead against mine. "Just this once, doll. Just this once—I will look toward tomorrow."

As if a needle scratches its mark to start a new song, the world halts after another monstrous blast.

A tsunami size wave of wind steals the gravity from beneath us. Like dominoes, we all fall from an invisible but all-powerful force. I squeeze my eyes, waiting for death to follow, but not without a finale to this terror.

A thunderous crack tears through the sky, and the speed of

sound breaks through the barrier, followed by a sonic blast. I want to press my palms against my ears, but I can't move. The world rumbles below my body, and I peek through cracks of my eyelids, scared to see what lies before me.

Thick black clouds are stealing every ounce of air and are closing in on me within its encumbrance. Everything is dark.

A steady ear-splitting ring vibrates through my head, replacing all other hints of sound.

The air wreaks of salt-ridden smoke and gunpowder, and the fumes fill my lungs.

I taste the soil and debris falling over me like snow on a lonely mountain top.

The record player ceases without a scratch.

There's nothing but a void.

20

DECEMBER 1941

THE RINGING in my ears is like static on the radio, with muffled voices trying to break through the airwaves. I press myself up to my knees, fighting off the dizzy weight holding me down. "Everett!" I try to shout but can't hear the sound coming from my mouth.

A dirt-covered hand sweeps across mine. The round cuticles and short nail beds with a freckle at the tip of his forefinger tell me it's Everett. It's hard to keep my eyes open within the thick smoke, but the warmth of his hand eases my overwhelming fear. I wish I knew how many more bombs those dive bombers are carrying. I want to know if they see us scampering, suffering, weak, and unable to move.

Everett pulls his hand away and his arm loops beneath my stomach, lifting me to my feet. His grip moves to my wrists. "It's the—zona." I can hardly make out every other word.

"I can't hear—" I cry out.

"The Arizona. It's gone."

With each second that passes, my ability to hear returns. The Arizona. Marines and Soldiers live onboard. I turn my neck to the side, looking out toward the harbor, but flames are engulfing the body of water. The smog has lifted enough to see the catastrophe unfolding before us, as if a sheet is slipping to the side a mangled, dead body.

Everett pulls me along the pier's edge, waving his hand and screaming above the various clashing pitches of resonance.

The words pouring from Everett's mouth emit in muddled howls, stinging my ears as he flags down one of the smaller vessels sailing toward us. A high-pitched scream in the distance pulls my attention away from the incoming vessel and out into the inky blazing waters. Arms flail. "So many of them are in the water. They are burning to their death," I say. I'm not sure if Everett hears me or has already seen what I'm witnessing, but he lowers me into the vessel as if I am a rag doll—a sailor taking me from Everett's grip. "Are you a civilian?" The man's words are clearer than anything else I've heard in the last few minutes.

"She's a nurse," Everett shouts from behind me, stepping into the boat. "Take her to the USS Solace. I'll help you pull bodies."

There isn't time for a formal introduction before the man grabs Everett's fist and helps him down onto the bilge of the vessel. "Billy Albert, Seaman First Class." Soot masks Billy's face and blonde sprigs of hair poke through the ashy layer of debris on his head. The whites of his eyes and the storm blue hues of his irises are all there is to see within the dark shadows of death cloaking his body.

"Everett Anderson, Lieutenant, Air Corps. This is Elizabeth Salzberg, Commander Salzberg's daughter." Their conversation is occurring as if we're standing on a sidewalk on a brilliant sunny day, rather than in a place where we should take cover from the bombers still flying above our heads. The thoughts of where Dad, James, and Lewis are burn through every blood vessel of my brain. Dad wouldn't have been on base at this hour on a Sunday, but he would receive a call at the first sight of the air raid. I don't know if there was enough time for him to make it to Ford Island. I pray there wasn't enough time. The last thing I said to him was, "... *how can you be so petulant and rude* ..." I will forever have to live with those horrible words spoken out of anger.

"I was on my way back to the ship when I heard the dive bombers coming for us. Before I knew it, I was asking myself why God would spare me after going home with this broad I met at the pub last night. I don't even know the girl's name, Anderson," Billy says with a choky laugh. How could he be carrying on a conversation like this right now? I can only assume he's in a state of shock.

Everett doesn't appear to be listening to what the guy is saying, but if he's a Seaman First Class, he might have seen Dad.

"Have you seen Commander Salzberg," I ask.

"Your old man?" Billy responds.

"I heard him over the radio before I took this vessel out to collect bodies."

The relief is slight, but it's substantial enough to allow some adrenaline to pump into my blood. I pray he kept James and Lewis safe, wherever they are.

Everett rests his hand on my knee and squeezes. "He's okay."

The men screaming for their lives in the water are not. "There's no time to drop me off at Solace. Let's grab some of these men," I say, leaning over the side. The heat raging from the bordering waters feels like a hot flash from diesel pluming out of the tailpipe of an old car.

"We won't be able to fit more than a few men into this lifeboat." How do we choose one life over another? There are so many men begging for help.

I wish the word "help" didn't have to sound like a breathless plea when the smog filled air is all that is keeping them alive and there doesn't seem to be enough to fill everyone's lungs.

Cries of pain sear through my blood as we reach the first oil-covered sailor. The grease is so thick I can't tell if he's wearing clothes or if the flames have burnt them off his body.

We reach for one of his two hands and pull him over the rim of the boat. "You're going to be okay," I say, pulling the sweater off my shoulders. "What's your name, sweetheart?" It's always the eyes that tell the story. Why does it have to be the one part of him I can see?

He's asking me a world of questions but hasn't moved his mouth since we dragged him into the boat. This look, the wide eyes searching mine for answers, the dilated pupils, and heavy breaths tell me there are significant injuries. "Freddy," he mumbles through gritted teeth.

"Freddy, can you tell me what hurts?" The more I inspect this man, the clearer I can see the breadth of damage to his skin. The oil is all he has protecting him, but it is also scorching and eating through every inch of his body.

"Everything," he mutters through a ferocious groan. If I touch him, it will feel like a thousand knives piercing his flesh and I don't have a stitch of medication to numb the pain.

"We're taking you to the USS Solace. We'll get you something for the pain as soon as we arrive. Do you want to squeeze my hand, Freddy?"

The screams of the next person we are heading to save grows louder than my voice. Freddy doesn't immediately respond, but as Everett and Billy are pulling in another body, Freddy takes my hand and squeezes with a weak grip. His hand is burning within mine and he clenches his eyes closed, crying tears from pain and fear.

"I don't want to die, Miss."

"Shh, no one is going anywhere. We're going to take care of you." Am I lying to this dying man? Is this what he should hear minutes before finding death? Fear is worse than pain, I know this. He needs hope to hold on to. "Freddy, can you tell me about your family? Do you have any sisters or brothers?"

With twitch-like movements, he nods his head. "A brother, Sam, and he's on the ship."

He's on the ship. The Arizona nearly submerged. "The Arizona?"

"Yes, Miss," he says, his words hard to hear as another wave of bomber planes dive over us.

"What about your parents?"

"Martha and Joe. We—we came from Texas. Just a small family and farm." Freddy's eyes roll from side to side as if confusion is setting in. "Where's Sam?" he cries out through agonizing gasps.

"Lizzie, we need you over here," Everett shouts while pressing his hands into a body's chest.

"Freddy, I'm going to ask you to hold on to my sweater for a minute while I go help another sailor out. I'll be right back."

"Sam!" Freddy shouts. "Sam, where are you? Answer me. Sam!"

I crawl across the rocking boat until I reach Everett's side. "He's not breathing."

I lean my ear toward the man's mouth, listening for the sound of airflow, but there's nothing. "Is there a pulse?" I press my finger into the side of his neck, searching for a carotid pulse. His eyes are wide open, staring up into the smoke-filled sky. "He's gone."

Everett runs his hand down to his mouth, gasping for air. "This is it, isn't it?"

"Don't talk like that. Do you hear me?"

"We can take one more man before we pull up to the Solace," Billy says.

"Lizzie, how are you so calm right now?" Everett asks.

"These men need us. What other choice is there? Go sit with Freddy. His brother was on the Arizona, and he doesn't know what the status of the ship is at the moment. Try to keep him distracted," I tell him, grabbing his shoulders to snap him out of the shock written along his face. "Look at me." I place my hand on his cheek. "This is why you are here. You're needed. God puts us where we should be."

Billy is trying to edge in close enough to the next guy, so I run to his side and grab a hand to pull the man up into the boat. Unlike Freddy and the other man, I see hints of white fabric covering his chest and there isn't a full covering of oil on his skivvies. He's covered from head to toe. "You're going to be okay, sweetheart. What's your name?"

"Keith Williamson. It's burning, Miss. Help me, please. Make it stop." I notice Keith has a contusion on the side of his head, the blood is hardly noticeable while mixed in with the black oil stains. I tear the hem of my dress and wrap the material around my hand to press to the side of his head. In response, Keith screams from the pressure of my hand. "I'm sorry, sweetie. We're almost to the hospital."

I check behind me, watching Everett talk to Freddy. Everett is pale, but his mouth is moving. He's doing what I said. I imagine the men going off to war must not entirely understand the reality they're about to face until it drops on them. I'm not positive any of us will survive today, but I can only look in front of us and keep going. Billy is steering us toward the boarding ramp of the Solace. Sailors are waiting by the open hatch of the ship with stretchers to help get these men off the boat, and I give them the scant rundown of information I have about the men. "This one here, he didn't make it."

Once the last of them are carried off the boat, I follow the sailors, stopping for a brief second in front of Everett. "I love you so much today, Everett. I've loved you every day before this one. And I'll love you for all of time—whatever that may be."

"I love you, always and forever, doll-face" he says, grabbing my hand. "Always and forever." I pull my hand from his, refusing to steal a moment of time from the men waiting for rescue.

The look on Everett's face says this is it. This is our last moment together and I don't know if one or both of us will die today, but the finality of our goodbye twists my stomach into a tight knot as I leap from the boat onto the ramp. I refuse to turn around. I can't. I don't want to see what goodbye looks like again.

"Where can I help? I'm a nurse," I shout to the entire flat area filled with double layered beds.

"Bed four," a nurse replies, pointing over her head. "Give him a shot of morphine for the burns. He's been in shock, unresponsive since he arrived." I inspect the man, wondering why the other nurses haven't cleaned them up at all, but the longer I think about the oil eating the skin off these men, I'm not sure we can clean them or have the time. "He'll be on the next transport to the hospital. He needs an amputation. Check the tourniquet every five minutes."

The nurse hasn't stopped shouting the list of injuries since I have arrived at this man's bedside. I pray he's sleeping and doesn't wake until this morphine kicks in. I inject the pain killer quicker than I would ever imagine doing, as if the man is dead. There's no reason for bedside manners or calming the patient down. The risk of infection is unthinkable with the oil dripping around the injection sight. I lift the sheet from the man's midsection, checking the tourniquet for spots of blood, but the gauze is still white. "He's stable, nurse," I reply.

"Bed eight, stop the bleeding." It doesn't take long to see how this nurse is keeping track of the patients. Every man brought in enters with an accompanying shout of assumed injury diagnosis. "We won't have enough morphine at this rate. Supplies will not last."

I was hoping there were more syringes and vials in the cart I pulled from. It was half full, half empty.

While I tend to bed eight, rounds of explosions throw the boat so hard the beds roll and swivels Piercing screams of pain erupt from every direction. "The last round of bombers hit more of our ships. A damn rescue vessel, too. I think they're coming back again too. Get down, get down," a voice screams out.

I don't know who is shouting the information, but I pull the bleeding man from his bed and use every ounce of strength in my body to push him beneath the bed. As we rock and slide to every single explosive thud, I search my surroundings for dressing to wrap this man's bleeding arm. "Don't worry about me, honey. I'll be okay," he says.

"We're all going to be okay; do you hear me? We're all going to be okay. I'm going to stop the bleeding on your arm. It may hurt a bit." The pain wouldn't have been as severe if the boat didn't sway so hard to the right. We're shielding ourselves from soaring unsecured objects. I'm doing my best to cover the man. "In case no one tells you today, Miss. You're a hero. You're my hero. Thank you."

A bomber plane hit a rescue vessel too. Was it my hero?

21

DECEMBER 1941

WHEN NOTHING ELSE MATTERS, when the only world I have ever known is gone, what difference do my actions make?

The ship stills, the rocking motion halts, and the deck is unnaturally quiet. "I'm going to help you back onto the bed now," I say to the patient, whose name I still don't know. "I need you to keep pressure on this arm while we move, okay?"

"Yes, Miss." I help the young man slide out along the slick floor. He's able to lift himself back onto the bed without using his left arm, which is bleeding through the towel he has pressed to the wound.

I don't know how many minutes have passed since Everett left with the rescue vessel to pick up more patients, but I know they can only fit five men in it at a time.

"Another incoming rescue vessel with patients is approaching," a sailor shouts from the port. "Prepare for triage."

We have several empty beds on this deck, but I know some men are making triage areas on other decks, too.

Please let this be Everett.

I'm trying to keep my focus on the patient I'm tending to, irrigating his wound to inspect for lodged shrapnel. The cut is clean from debris, just deep and wide. "This will need sutures," I tell him. "We need the bleeding to slow down first, so I'm going to need your help keeping pressure on the towel."

"Yes, Miss, but you aren't going far, right?"

"I need to help the incoming patients, but I'll back in just a moment to check on you. You're going to be just fine. Don't you worry, sweetheart."

Bile rises from the barren depths of my stomach as I race toward the port to help the incoming men with injuries. The rescue groups have lined up stretchers, ready for patients on the short loading ramp. The rescue vessel preparing for transport is different from the one I arrived in. There are three men helping the injured, not two. None of them are Everett.

"How many men were on the rescue vessel that went down?" A sailor shouts out to the waters.

"We don't know yet. It's gone."

"Gone as in—"

"It blew up. It's gone and we can't focus on that right now. One of these men has minutes left, maybe less. I need to get him in there first. Let's go. Come on," I hear from outside. "He's not breathing, but he has a slow pulse. The explosion stole both his legs."

Everett is still alive.

I must believe.

He has to be okay.

I must focus on these men who need care.

Everything is going to be all right. It must be.

As I help them with the stretcher, everything around me seems to move in slow motion while I focus my thoughts on where they should be. "There are four more rescue vessels behind us, filled with severely injured men. How many beds do you have left?"

"We don't have many beds at all, a dozen at most. We need to transfer the critical to the hospital."

"Stabilize those men so we can move them."

The conversation continues and the orders keep coming.

There are four more rescue vessels approaching.

There are too many injured men to care for here.

We need to stabilize the critical and move them out of her as fast as possible.

Every nurse on this ship is elbow deep in blood and burning

oil. Patients are screaming, crying, pleading for mercy. I find the man who's dying and begin a set of chest compressions while a medic wraps his legs. "Come on. Stay with me," I chant mindlessly as I use every ounce of strength to press the heels of my hands into his chest. He looks so young, maybe just eighteen. He's not ready to die. I close my eyes and forget the exhaustion wreaking havoc on my arms. "Come on. Breathe."

Five minutes pass and there's still the slightest sensation of a pulse. There is still hope. It seems as if there are more injured men arriving every time I turn around. The moans and cries grow louder than the shouting orders. "We need to move onto the next bed," a doctor says from behind me. "You've done all you can do."

"No," I shout, pressing harder and firmer into the man's chest.

Water expels from his mouth as if shooting from a spout. I tilt his head to the side, allowing the water to spill off his face. He coughs and gags on the oil-laced liquid as more comes up. There is little color on the man's cheeks, but his eyes open. I place my fingers on the side of his neck, finding his pulse stronger and faster. "You're going to be okay," I tell him.

"There are no more beds," a sailor shouts from an open hatch. "We're running out of supplies too. We need to get these men over to the hospital."

"It's not safe to transport them yet. Those damn dive bombers are still out there ready to drop another load," a man hollers from a deck above ours.

I thought it was over. I was praying they ran out of ammunition, bombs, torpedoes, and whatever else they're trying to murder us with. How many more explosions will we survive?

"Help!" The scream is shrill. Panic is raw and raging through the deck, like a hurricane. These men must know the attack is far from over. None of the less critical patients are focusing on the pain writhing through their bodies. Some of them are dressing each other's wounds because we aren't making our rounds fast enough. There aren't enough of us.

I search for the source of crying pleas, finding Freddy in the corner. Parts of his face are clear of the burning oil, but in its place is raw flesh. I flee to his side. "I'm here, I'm here, Freddy." I inspect him to gauge where the pain is escalating from, but no sooner do I open my mouth to ask what's changed that I spot the evidence beneath his fingernails. He scratched the oil off his face along with the top layer of skin. I'm living in a horror picture, a well scripted one. I'm not one to get queasy at anything except the sight of vomit, which I have tried hard to overcome the last several months, but the sheer look of agony and the gruesome wounds are gutting me.

"Why won't the burning stop?" Freddy continues to shout. "Make it stop!"

"Okay, I'm going to apply more petroleum jelly, but I need you to remain still." I lean forward, inching my stare closer to his, hoping to capture his full attention. The sound of explosions erupting seems further away than it was. I can only hope the Japanese have run out of ammunition and bombs.

"Miss, I want to go home. I just want to go home. Will you help me find Sam and take him home too. Please, please," he cries out. "He's my big brother—the best big brother any guy could ask for. Sam enlisted because I did. He wanted to watch over me. What if he's gone? What will I tell our parents? This is my fault. It's all my fault. Help me, please." His questions and statements are like hundreds of fishhooks, gutting me alive. I haven't heard anything about his missing brother. He could be in one of these beds, still drowning, or shredded in body parts at the bottom of the ocean.

"Freddy, I want to help you get home, Sam too. Tell me your last name, sweetheart."

"Winthrop," he mutters. "Our names are Frederick Winthrop and my brother, Samuel. We need to get home."

"Sir, I need to advise you to sit back down. You are in no shape to go fight," a nurse scolds a patient behind me. I twist my head over my shoulder, spotting a man with burns and minor contusions. His burns are far less severe than Freddy's. I'm betting it's because of the uniform he's wearing beneath the oil. Those who were asleep in their barracks on the ship were only in their skivvies, and they are the ones suffering the most. Anyone in uniform may have been spared from the worst of it. At least that's how it looks from what I can see on this deck.

"It is my duty and right to defend our men and country. And with all due respect Ma'am, the probability of us being the next target is just as likely as me sustaining additional injuries out there. I need to defend. They need me."

"No, you have serious injuries. The water is contaminated, and you will get yourself an infection," the nurse argues.

"Let him go," I shout. "We're all doing what we can to save each other. If he saves one person along with himself, he's done more out there than in here."

I'm aware that I'm speaking out of turn. I don't work on this ship, nor do I belong on this ship, but I can't watch these men die without a fighting chance, and if there's anything I can do to save even one life, I will do it regardless of what anyone thinks. The middle-age nurse seems taken aback by my remark but doesn't respond.

"You're a smart gal," the sailor says to me, jumping from his cot.

Four others in the vicinity stand up, two still bleeding, one with burns covering half of his upper torso. "We're going too. If they're dying out there, we're all dying together."

The older nurse slaps her hands against her sides. "This is preposterous. You, gentlemen have injuries and need medical attention. You're risking your lives."

"That's what we do, Ma'am. We're here to risk our lives. Now, if you please, pardon us."

The five men don't wait for a response. They don't wait for a rescue vessel. One by one, they dive back into the waters, ready to dodge bullets and recover more men. "What on earth gives you the right to step in front me at a time like this? I don't even know who you are," the nurse says, stepping in front of me with abruptness.

"I'm Commander Salzberg's daughter, Elizabeth Salzberg, a certified nurse, and I'm helping the best I can, going above and beyond the responsibilities of my civilian duties. We are all losing a battle here today, Ma'am, and if you don't allow these men to do what they have been trained to do, then you will spend more time fighting with patients today than you will saving their lives. Forgive my crass tone, but we are all in this together and there isn't a moment to second guess or spare. We are here to help the wounded, not hold them against their will because of rules that didn't consider the tragedy we are witnessing today."

The nurse, who looks to have years of experience above mine, looks appalled by my comments. Her eyes are wide, stained with red veins—a look of shock tugging at every fine line encasing her mouth. "I didn't realize who you were. My apologies."

I never admit to who I am—being a commander's daughter, but if the power of my last name has any leverage for good use, I will use it in the way Dad would. "Apologies aren't necessary. We are running low on morphine. If we cannot evacuate these men soon, do you know if we have a supply drop coming in?"

The woman continues to stare at me, as if in traumatic shock —as if this is the first moment reality has begun to strangle her. She wraps her hands around my arms. "You're right, Miss Salzberg. You're a brilliant young woman. We need supplies. I will call for supplies." The color in her cheeks fades to a dull pink. *She's recalling the last hour of our lives, the images she will never forget.*

At this moment, I'm not sure any of us will ever see another sunset.

22

DECEMBER 1941

THE HOSPITAL IS at its capacity, injured men fill every available cot, and each spare chair is warm. Supply runs are occurring more frequently, and the cries are becoming softer. We work as the minutes blend into the afternoon hours while writing out the names of men who didn't survive—those who died in our presence, in agony, struggling for breaths, and wishing to see their families once more. I watched the time run out again and again, and I was the recipient of last words, final prayers, pleading wishes, and messages in need of reaching the proper recipients. I found a small notebook in the supply closet, and I've been keeping track of the names of those who made requests.

For all the soldiers and sailors recovering from an amputation, or losing multiple missing limbs, they lay in their cots, staring at the ceiling, as they imagine a future without part of their past.

The burn victims—most of the critically wounded are still in a state of sedation, mute, numb, and unknowing. Forever, they will remain scarred by the horrors of today. Each time they look in a mirror, they will replay the pain of wishing for death over life, and the reminder of the moment they lost their identity.

We're still missing so many men. The columns on lists are accumulating, all information on display publicly for those searching for a loved one.

I'm looking for my loved ones.

During the brief moments I'm able to take a breath, I realize I haven't exchanged words with a familiar face since arriving at the hospital just before noon. Red Cross nurses have arrived to assist, but across the base, there are less than a hundred nurses aiding what we think to be nearly one thousand injured men. However, the more recent tallies are showing over two thousand casualties. There are more deaths than those hanging onto a sliver of life, and I don't recognize even one of the tormented souls lying around me.

With my round of patients stable for the moment, I step into the corridor, lined with military personnel and civilians finding debris and black soot covering everyone and every object. It's not surprising to see since I have been coughing for hours, trying to clear my lungs from what I inhaled. My chokes are minimal, if not insignificant compared to the haunting gasps for air echoing through the halls. The sounds follow me as I try to move at a quick pace, but my legs are heavy, like I'm carrying the weight of life and death on my shoulders.

I push my sleeves up above my elbows, desperate to cool down, but the sight of my skin exposes more blood stains and oil. I'm covered.

The devastation is overwhelming.

My muscles ache, my heart is throbbing, and I want to fall to the ground and cry for every lost soul. But I can't. There's no time to look back.

I will not allow this attack to take us all down. I have to focus on the path in front of me and block out the rest, my sole purpose being to save a part of humanity and our country.

"My life matters less," Mom always told me, referring to herself. *"For, life isn't worth living, unless we devote our blessings to others in need. When everyone gives, we all receive. Each of us is here for a reason, one written in the stars on the day we were born."*

Mom's voice and viewpoints made me want to become a journalist, but her actions spoke louder than her words, and I need to continue her path of giving, both out of respect to her memory and my conscience.

I'm not sure if my actions from today are noble because there were too many instances that I had to ignore procedure and protocol, temporarily mending wounds to make cots available for others. I felt as though I was trading one life for another.

"Elizabeth!" I recognize the voice but can't place it to a face among the agonizing harmony of moans and groans. "Elizabeth Salzberg, is that you?" I peer in every direction, searching for a familiar person among the crowd of calamity before I spot her face.

Nurse Jones, my teacher and mentor who carried me through my nursing certification. "I didn't know you were here." She walks as if the pain in her legs mirrors mine. Her arms reach out and pull me in tightly against her broad chest.

I squeeze my eyes, unsure If I deserve the warmth of her embrace when the fires of Hell are raging around me. I see a woman who wore me to the bone many days over the last few years, and who was never afraid to scold me when I made a mistake. She never put me on a pedestal for being a commander's daughter. If anything, she was harder on me for it, but also gave me the foundation to grow and told me I was unstoppable. She pleaded with me to take the position at this hospital over moving to Boston. I still hadn't given her my answer. Now, I don't know what my future holds. Nurse Jones will not release her hold around my arms. "Are you okay?" I ask.

As the words slip from my mouth, I realize how ridiculous the question is. Of course she's not okay.

"Thank goodness you are here and you're safe," she says. "Your father has been calling here every half hour to check the list for your name. I did not know you were working in a unit. I've been in triage all day."

I glance toward the front entrance of the hospital where the list is; it's as if the list is another enemy chasing after all of us.

"I was in the wrong place at the right time. I started at the Solace and made my way over here around noon," I tell her.

"Please stay," she pleads.

"I'm not going anywhere, Nurse Jones. I will stay until I tend to all necessary injuries."

Nurse Jones takes a step back and claws her long nails around my chin. "You are unstoppable, like I've always told you. Never look back, Elizabeth. Keep going. You hear me?"

"Yes, Ma'am."

"What ward are you circulating?"

I point down the endless looking corridor. "ICU, unit three, block two."

Nurse Jones pats me on the shoulder. "I'm not surprised they placed you there. I'll check in with you shortly."

With a single nod, I continue moving forward, but she takes my arm and twists me around. "Thank you, Elizabeth. Thank you."

Gratitude isn't necessary when so many are lying around me, maimed or dead.

I walk to the board, perusing the list of names that are now in categories of casualty type, including those who were dead on arrival. It will take too long to read through all the names, so I try to convince myself that since I don't see Everett's name in D.O.E. column, it must be good news. Surely, his name would stand out amongst the rest.

* * *

Another round of antibiotics, pain relievers, ointments, and intravenous drops leaves me weak. My eyes are burning, I've been short of breath for hours, and my stamina is waning. I grip the metal bar of the rolling cart of supplies and grit my teeth so hard, pain radiates through my jaw.

I have to keep going.

They're depending on me.

"Nurse Salzberg, a moment please," I hear from the other end of the block of cots. I press up on my toes to see between the beds and patients, finding Nurse Jones summoning me with a wave of her hand. She steps out between the curtains separating two blocks in the unit. I brush the sweat-laced hair from my forehead while turning the corner.

"Yes, Nurse Jones. I just completed the third round of morphine for beds one through ten."

When she moves out of my direct line of sight, I see Dad standing in front of me, paler than a ghost, and disheveled like I've never seen. A man who only shows emotion through his eyes is quivering at the chin. His chest lurches as a heavy sob bellows between us. He reaches for me and yanks me to him with what must be all the remaining strength in his body.

"My baby," he cries. "I thought I lost you today. I thought I lost you, Elizabeth. I can't lose you. Do you understand? I can't lose you."

"I heard your name echoing through the halls today, confirming your status, but I didn't know where you were," I reply.

He's holding me so tightly I'm having trouble breathing, forcing me to cough up the putrid taste of what I assume gasoline fumes, oil residue, and gun powder taste like. Dad presses his hands down onto my shoulders and pushes me back a step.

"Have you been assisting all day?"

"Yes, I was at the Solace until noon, then evacuated to the hospital. They needed help."

There's a look in his eyes, not of anger, frustration, or grief. The expression doesn't match the darkness of our environment. He's blacking the world out, focusing on just me.

"She would be so proud of you right now," he mutters. "I see so much of your mother in you and she is living through your eyes today, Elizabeth. You are everything she dreamed you would be."

I will not cry. I will not give my tears to the enemy. Words are weaker than actions. They are only sounds. I have her strength. That's what he sees. I swallow the lump in my throat and stare straight back into Dad's eyes.

"Mom carved a path I couldn't ignore." Dad brings me back in against his chest again, holding the palm of his hand behind my head. "Where are James and Lewis?"

"They're safe," Dad says. "They've been searching for you all day too. No one knew where you were."

I nod through his tight hold. "I'm thankful you're okay. I knew you would be," I say.

"I didn't—I wasn't sure of anything today," he says.

I pull away from his embrace and inhale sharply, pushing away the stabbing pain in my chest. "I have a lot of patients waiting on me."

"I don't want to keep you." Dad runs his hands over his chin, staring past me for a moment. "Elizabeth, I don't want you to go home tonight. I'm not sure when I will be off duty, or your brothers. Will you stay here? I believe it's safest."

"Yes, Dad."

"I love you, Elizabeth—with all my heart and soul." Dad reaches for my neck and slips the necklace chain out from beneath my collar. "I was wrong. Wear this as a symbol of who you are. Be proud. It isn't time to hide. It's time to rise above the ashes."

When the necklace hits the outside of my collar, I clutch my hand over the gold star, holding it as if it has the power to make everything better.

"I love you too, Dad."

He's still staring at me as if he has something left to say but can't find the words. I'm afraid of whatever secrets are hiding behind his half-lidded, tired eyes.

"Have you heard anything about Everett's status?"

Dad's head bows, breaking his eye contact with me. "Elizabeth, I—I'm—"

"Nurse Elizabeth, cot four in unit two is bleeding out," someone shouts.

"Go take care of your patient. Everything will be okay. You must stay focused right now. Their lives depend on it," he says, pointing toward the curtain behind me.

"Dad?"

While holding a truth that could break my world into a million pieces, he walks away as I hear my name once again. I'm left with Mom's words, "My life matters less." It's a painful strike of the chords in my heart.

23

DECEMBER 1941

HOW CAN I sleep knowing today will become a yesterday I will want to forget—a yesterday that holds a goodbye I will need to hold on to forever?

I know why Dad ran off without offering a response about Everett. He mustn't think I've forgotten his logic for dealing with a situation such as this.

August 1933

I was twelve, hardly old enough to understand the catastrophes that can unfold during a naval deployment. It wasn't the first time Dad had to leave us for some time to uphold his civic duties, but it was the first time his eyes revealed a deep, weary thought. I must have asked him if everything was all right at least a dozen times in the days prior to his departure.

The night before he was to report for duty on the ship, he knocked on my bedroom door and strolled in with his hands tucked into his pockets and a fake smile etched into his rigid jaw.

"Do you have a moment for your old man?" Dad asked.

If I remember correctly, I was in the middle of counting the brush strokes through a section of my golden hair. "I always have time for you, Daddy."

He nudged his head, silently hinting for me to scoot over in my bed. It had been a while since he had sat with me until I fell asleep or read me a story. I was teetering on the timeline of becoming a teenager, a daughter who no longer needed her daddy to tuck her in every night. He sat on top of the folded sheet, resting his legs down on the royal blue quilt. "I need to ask you a big favor, sweetheart."

"Do you need me to pick up your mail or deliver any important letters to anyone while you're gone?" I always wanted an assignment or a role to feel like I was taking part in the important work Dad did.

"No, no, nothing like that, Elizabeth. I need to ask that you mind your mother and help her around the house. Your brothers are getting older now and they're both going to continue working throughout the school year in addition to playing on the football team. Things might be a little chaotic here while I'm not home."

"I'm sure we'll all be just fine, Daddy. There's nothing you need to worry about."

Dad twists his head, giving me a look paired with a raised brow. "My youngest child who searches for adventure on cliffs and in shark-ridden waters, rebels against housework, and referred to as 'too-wild-to-tame' by many of our neighbors, is telling me I have nothing to worry about," he said with a chuckle.

I sat up taller against my pillow. "You can't blame me for being a curious girl who wants to see every inch of the world. Did you know that there are more inches from one side of the globe to the other than there are minutes in a person's lifetime?"

"Well, now that all depends on what path you take and how long you live, young lady."

"Only with shortcuts," I argued.

"Elizabeth, I'm going to be on a warship heading to Guantanamo Bay per orders of the president. Without getting into too much detail, I need to leave here with peace of mind, knowing you are going to be safe and helping your mother rather than making her chase you like a loose goose. When I worry about what is happening at home, I can't focus on my tasks as clearly as I need to be. You, your brothers, and your mother are always on my mind, but I need a sense of contentment to fill those thoughts. If a man is worried about the life he left at home, he will be the first to fall during a battle. I've seen it happen time and time again."

"I don't want anything bad to happen to you, daddy. You know I'll do everything I can to help mom and do what she says—I promise."

"That's all I can ask, sweetheart. Thank you for understanding." With

a sigh of relief, Dad placed a kiss on my cheek and tucked me into bed. "I'll wake you up to say goodbye before I leave in the morning."

When the lights went out and the door closed, his words replayed in my head: "If a man is worried about the life he left at home, he will be the first to fall during a battle. I've seen it happen time and time again." I couldn't understand how anyone could block out their life during a deployment.

Now I see ... if *a woman* is worried about a man she loves, she will be the first to fail at saving another's life.

I set up a chair between the draped blocks filled to the brim with critically injured men. Most are asleep or in a daze from the drugs, and I have an hour before I need to make my rounds unless someone calls for me before then. It might be my only opportunity to get a little shut eye. The discomfort of a straight l-shaped wooden chair can't compete with the heaviness of my eyelids. I rest my head against the wall and try to focus on anything but what I've witnessed in the last fourteen hours.

* * *

"Pardon me, Miss."

I'm startled as my eyes flash open, finding a tattered man with sad eyes standing before me. Once my vision clears, the memories jog back to this morning or yesterday. I'm not sure if it's after midnight yet, but I surely should have woken by now. I glance at my wristwatch, noting the time to be five minutes before midnight.

"It's me, Billy Albert. I picked you up on the rescue vessel this morning."

I place my hand against the side of my face, wondering why I didn't recognize him right away. The number of faces, or lack thereof, I have seen today are blending.

"Billy, goodness ... are you all right?" I ask, standing up while rubbing away the exhaustion from beneath my eyes.

"Yes, Miss. I will be okay, physically. How are you?"

"Do you know where Everett is?" If Billy is alive and they

were together after leaving me at the Solace, surely their vessel wasn't the one that took the hit.

"He isn't here?"

My eyebrows furrow in response to his question. "Why would he be here?"

Billy shakes his head. "I'm not sure where he went. He was yelling about something when he took off at a pier. I figured he'd gone looking for you since we couldn't get back over to the Solace easily after the second round of attacks."

My gaze drops to the blood-stained floor. "I don't know where he would be."

Billy presses his soot covered fingers beneath my chin, forcing me to look up at him. "Don't give up hope, Miss Salzberg."

Multiple groans and moans grow from the ICU block. "The morphine is wearing off," I explain.

"We're grateful for you. I need to go update the list of casualties. Take care of yourself, Miss Salzberg. I promise to keep my sights out for Lieutenant Anderson."

I wrap my arms around his neck for a quick embrace, feeling him wince beneath my grip. "Please get yourself checked out, Billy."

"I'm just sore. Don't worry about me."

"Thank you for the wake-up call," I say, offering a small smile.

He tips his head and pivots on his heels to leave in the opposite direction.

I gather a cart of supplies for the rounds, preparing several doses of morphine to administer first. Some dressings need checking, and any blood loss from the amputees. Other than the most severely injured, most of the others are stable at the moment, aside from pain, but infection can set in rapidly if we don't monitor their wounds closely. Once we make it past the point of infection, morale will be what counts more than the pain killers.

"Miss, could you do me a favor when you have a moment?" a gentleman from a bed across the block asks.

"Yes, Sir. What can I do for you?"

"Could you check the list for a name?"

After noting how long the list was earlier, I have been avoiding the idea of looking at it again. "Of course, Sir. What's the name?"

"Danny Paige. He's my brother."

"I'm happy to go look just as soon as I finish checking on the rest of the men here."

I haven't had to inform anyone of a death. I pray his brother's name isn't on there, but as I know well, it doesn't quite matter if his name is or isn't on the list. There are so many men still unaccounted for.

"He was on The Arizona." I glance at the man's file in search of his name. Trevor Paige. He also was on The Arizona, but one of the least injured of what I've seen today.

I find myself in a fog as I move to the next bed, realizing I'm allowing my emotions to slip ahead of my focus. I squeeze my eyes tightly, swallow hard and take in a deep breath. This man is most important now. There is no one else.

Gunnery Sergeant Peters is one of the few soldiers I've had in this block. Most of the injured have been sailors. He's awake but lost in his mind, staring at the white speckled ceiling.

"How are you feeling, Gunnery Sergeant?" I ask, placing my hand on his shoulder. He doesn't flinch or blink. His cheeks are pale and dewy, and when I check his pulse, I find a rapid heartbeat along with short, quick breaths. "Can you hear me, Gunnery Sergeant?"

Still no response. He's in shock, but there could be a dozen different reasons for his trance-like expression. The dressing around the capped amputation of his right arm is burgundy and nowhere near as tight as it should be, or as I left it earlier. Blood is oozing from the wound. It wasn't before. I increase the flow of IV fluids and tend to the dressing on the wound, finding the pale pallor of his skin morphing into a gray hue toward his elbow.

"Gunnery Sergeant, could you blink if you hear me talking?"

Nothing. I should have been watching him more closely. This is my fault.

"He loosened the tourniquet, nurse. I watched him do it," the patient in the next bed over states. I look back and forth between the man speaking and the patient I'm treating, wondering why he would do such a thing. "We've seen too much. I can't say I blame him for wanting to give up."

Give up. The words sear through my stomach.

I grab a belt tourniquet from my cart and place it above the stump, pulling the soft leather with all the strength I have. The sling hanging from the metal bar above needs to be higher to assist the blood flow to the proper direction.

"I need a medic in Unit 2, Block A, Bed 5," I shout. "Hemorrhage." The color isn't returning to his skin and his pulse is still racing. The medic who has been making his rounds through this unit for most of the day brushes by the draped curtains. "He may need a transfusion."

"Yes, go ahead," the medic instructs before leaving as swiftly as he arrived.

This man's life is in my hands, and if I'm wrong, he could die. He could end up being another name on the list.

24

DECEMBER 1941

THE LIST IS endless and growing.

I'm dizzy, weak, and feeling unstable on my feet. One of the head nurses in the hospital told me to take a break, but there's nowhere to go. The gateway between the destruction outside and the ever-expanding list of names enshrouds me — my world — what was my world.

I've tried to phone Audrey's house, but there is no answer. For all I know, our street may not exist anymore. I hope she and her family are safe. Any attempt at feeling hopeful seems futile with the numbers rising so rapidly.

I walk toward the front doors, finding momentary solace at the sight of the wavering palm leaves, but seeing the abundance of wreckage, including a wing of a Japanese bomber plane — just a wing, snaps my mind back to reality.

The air is thick with dust and fumes, disrupting the typical visibility of the surrounding area. I pull my collar up over my mouth and nose to block the acrid cloud of smoke. A convoy of military and civilian vehicles advance through the base as if they are in sync with one another, leaving a space of three feet in front and three feet behind each set of wheels.

"Miss, you can't be out here. You must evacuate immediately."

"Evacuate?" I question the soldier marching toward me.

"Yes, we are currently under martial law. All civilians are to evacuate the base for their safety. I'll help you into a vehicle."

"I beg your pardon, Sir, but I am not going anywhere. There are men under my care inside this hospital and I cannot simply leave per your terms."

The soldier scans my attire from head to toe. "My apologies, Miss, but you aren't in uniform."

"There wasn't time to change my clothes," I inform the man.

"It isn't safe out here. Please step back inside the hospital."

I want to put this man in his place for speaking to me the way he did, but more importantly, I would like to ask him if he has lived through the same twenty-four hours I have? Has he learned anything? At the very least, it should have taught him the proper way to speak to someone. The possibility of martial law has been brought up many times. It has been a backup plan if or when the United States were to be under attack during the war. The military shall handle all laws now. We, the people, will essentially lose our freedom. The safest thing for me to do would be to run and hide, but I will not leave, certainly not by the words of this soldier

"How are we supposed to go about finding loved ones?"

"I don't have a proper answer to your question at the moment. I'm sure they will brief us on reconnecting families soon."

"Very well," I say, turning my back to him so I can head to the hospital.

"If I find you out here again, I will have to escort you to an evacuation vehicle. This is no place for a woman to be standing around. Surely, you understand the danger we're facing."

I close my eyes and tug in a quick breath before turning back to face the young man. "I should truly bite my tongue, soldier, but in good conscience to myself, I cannot. Those of us who are still alive have been through the direst circumstances one could ever imagine. I was unaware of the instatement of Martial Law since I was tending to the wounded victims and trying to save lives inside the hospital. That's what I did after enduring the second wave of air raid attacks in the moments that followed my departure from the USS Solace. My clothes are covered in blood from many people. There is a lack of fresh air inside the hospital, and the only

scent permeating the building is that of bile and death. I have
been caring for the casualties since yesterday morning and needed
to find a breath of cleaner air. I failed miserably since there was
none outside either, but I will take a break when I need one and
your newfound control will not threaten me."

"Ma'am, I—I understand—" he stutters, looking visibly
shaken by my words.

"I won't ask you where you were yesterday at seven in the
morning because it doesn't matter. This island—our country is not
a safe place for women or men right now, but if it weren't for the
women inside of that building, there would many more dead
men."

"Yes, Ma'am, And I thank you for your service."

"And I thank you for yours. Please, do not confuse following
orders for being rude and disrespectful. We are all in this
together."

The soldier dips his head toward me and I take the moment to
walk away, leaving silence in my place. It would have been
simpler to inform the man who my father is then giving him a
lesson on honor and respect, but I'm tired of using my last name
as a crutch. If we, as a nation, don't handle this moment properly,
it will define humanity possibly forever and I will not be a part of
that.

I return to the foyer of the hospital, once again facing the
updated list of those injured or dead. As requested, I have perused
the board several times without stumbling over Everett or
Audrey's names, but not seeing their names on the list only gives
me momentary relief since there are other field hospitals set up
around the base. There are a dozen locations for the injured, and
many of the patients are unidentifiable, as I've seen.

"I thought I told you to go take a break." Nurse Rose
approaches me from a blind spot around the corner. "We have you
covered for a couple hours now that more of the Red Cross nurses
have arrived."

"I know. It's just better to keep moving right now," I explain.
If I take a seat, I'm not sure I'll be able to get back up so easily.

"Go clean yourself up, put on a uniform. Coffee and food will
help too. We need you, Nurse Salzberg."

We're in the middle of a war, a battle we're not winning. People don't take breaks while under fire. "I'll be back in just a few minutes."

I follow a trail of blood toward the stairwell, wondering if the remnants are from one person or many. I veer away from the scarlet stains out of respect and descend twelve steps to the next level down.

"Excuse me, could you help me locate Nurse Salzberg," I hear a muffled voice from around the corner holding me frozen in place between a set of tiled walls.

"I believe she was heading to the nurse's quarters."

My body feels heavy, as if weighed down by cement, and I can't move. "Lizzie."

I try to inhale but my throat tightens, my eyes widen, and I clutch my chest as I turn toward the voice. He's nearly unrecognizable, his clothes are soaking wet, sticking to his skin. His hands are black with dirt and oil. His face has smudges of grease and soot, and his hair is falling over his left eye.

"You're alive," I whisper as a statement rather than a question, but I feel the need to reach out and touch him, so I'll know I'm not hallucinating.

"I'm sorry I couldn't find you sooner."

My eyes strain and ache as I refuse to blink. I cup my hand over my mouth, holding back the sob quaking through my chest. Everett reaches forward and takes my wrist in his hand, tugging me in toward him. He presses the side of my face against his chest and loops his free arm around my back, holding me firmly within his trembling grip.

"I didn't know if you made it here, but I crossed paths with your father about an hour ago. He thought I hadn't made it off the tugboat."

"You're here," I mutter against his wet shirt.

"I was so scared, Lizzie. I'm still scared. We only had a few planes left, and I was too late by the time I got to the airfield. I found weapons and fired until ammunition ran low. I don't know if it was all in vain. Then I helped rescue more of the trapped men on the ships. So many more died than those rescued."

I squeeze my arms around his torso, wishing there was a way to be closer than we already are. "Are you hurt?"

He rests his cheek on the top of my head. "Just a couple of burns and superficial scratches. I'm fine. Are you okay?"

What is the definition of being okay? "Physically, yes, I'm fine."

"I can't stay here, doll-face. I'm on duty and supposed to report to the captain at zero-nine-hundred, but I needed to find you first."

"I understand," I say, swallowing hard against my aching throat.

"I will come back for you tonight. Don't leave the hospital. We have activated martial law and must evacuate all civilians from base."

I want to tell him I'm scared too but hearing those words would do him no good. There's no guarantee I'm safe here in the hospital or if it's any safer outside, but we don't know what life has in store for use beyond this hour. "Please don't leave," I beg. There's a sudden vulnerability I've never shown him before. I've always wanted him to see me as an equal—strong and independent, but everything is different now and I can't hold back my feelings. "I know that once you walk away, I'll wonder if this moment was real or if I'm hallucinating from sheer exhaustion. Everett, I'm not sure how much more I can take." I've never sounded so subdued and unpretentious, but I want to hold on to him now more than ever. I know it's not possible, though. Feeling safe and content is no longer within reach for either of us.

"Look at me, doll," he says, slipping his finger beneath my chin.

I tilt my head back to glance up into his eyes. His gaze appears unfocused, as if he can't see anything but what is directly in front of him. The memories of what he witnessed will remain crisp and clear, never erased by time. I don't know if we will get to see life as it used to be—light and carefree, like a warm, tropical breeze, or if images of the horror branded into our brains will overshadow every future thought. I place my hands on his cheeks, feeling the day-old stubble tickle the insides of my palms.

"I can only see pain. Is that all that's left for us?" I ask.

Everett shakes his head. "No, Lizzie, you shouldn't talk that way. We're both still here, and we're going to make it through this. Do you hear me?"

"What if it isn't over?" I question. I knew the moment I let the fear seep into my brain, it would suffocate me entirely. "What if this isn't real? Maybe I'm already dead and this is our last goodbye. Is that possible?"

"Shh," Everett hushes me, sweeping a strand of hair away from my forehead. "You aren't dead. I'm not dead. Everything will be okay. You'll see."

"I want to believe you more than I've ever believed anything in my life," I say, my voice croaking as a testament of exhaustion.

"You must," he says, placing a kiss on my cheek. "You need to have faith." I squeeze my arms around his back, coaxing a quiet groan from the bottom of his throat. "I will be back as soon as I can."

A tear escapes the corner of my eye and spills down the side of my cheek, but I swat at it with the back of my hand as if the weakness is a sign of surrendering. "Are you sure you are okay, Everett?"

He leans down and touches his lips to mine, inhaling sharply, then holds his breath for a long second. I would give him all the air in my lungs if I could. "I am now."

For the first time in the longest day I have lived, my body fills with a hint of warmth, protection, and safety.

"I love you, Lizzie, always and forever."

"I love you too, Everett."

He pulls back gently, releasing the hold I have on him, leaving me without his tender heart to lean on or the comfort I feel when I'm in his arms. I reach my arms back toward him to hold on for a few more seconds, but his gaze drops to my hand clenching his. His forehead wrinkles as he covers his hand over his eyes. "I'm sorry I have to leave you again, Lizzie, but I have to go now."

I release my hand, wanting to fall to the ground and weep until the pain oozes out of every pore of my body.

"Goodbye, my love," I mutter through a weak breath.

"I'll be back. I promise, baby."

He's gone, leaving me with only a cool draft in the empty

corridor. I lean back against the wall, shivering from the loss of hope I felt for a brief few minutes.

* * *

It took me a bit to pick myself up and refocus my attention on what should have been a break to clean myself up.

As I approach the nurse's quarters, I find only a few other nurses in the room, and no one is speaking. They seem to be here for the same reason I am; to remove the remnants of death from their bodies by donning clean garments.

There is a pile of laundered uniforms in the corner, so I lift one off the table. The scent of bleach and detergent wafting around my nose takes me back to a few days prior, when I was doing Dad's and the boys' laundry at home. Life was so simple. I just didn't know it before yesterday.

"Have either of you seen Nurse Audrey Evans?" I ask.

The women both shake their heads in unison. "No, sweetie, we're both from the Red Cross. I'm afraid we don't know many of the staff here yet."

"Of course," I respond. Audrey took an offered position here just a month after we completed our training. She had her mind set on what would come next for her. She was clear about the fact that her life is here, and she will remain on this base.

With the folded linen pinched between my hands, I head down the hallway toward the powder room. In moments like this, when there is no one around and silence consumes me, I question every decision I made between yesterday morning and today. I base my decisions on gut instinct rather than taking time to mull things over.

I place the clean uniform on the base of the sink and twist the nozzle on the faucet, watching the water fire out in bursts for a few quick seconds before a steady stream flows into the basin. I fill my hands with soap and lean over the sink to wash my face, rubbing the soap into my eyes during a moment of distraction. The burn numbs my thoughts for a few moments. I need more of that. The cool water sends chills through my nerves and I rub at my cheeks, nose, forehead, and chin as tersely as I can stand to scrape away the remnants of someone's last moments. I continue scratching at my skin with the length of my fingernails, wiping away the grime from my arms and neck. My nail beds are a rusty-brown and there is dirt caked beneath the tips. I have been avoiding my reflection, refusing to give into the reality of what my eyes will now see in the mirror—a broken woman who has seen too much and comprehends the meaning of loss more than she should.

"*You are stronger than you realize,*" Mom always told me. "*Keep fighting, Elizabeth. We Salzberg women do not give up.*"

Recalling Mom's words forces me to see myself in a different light. My pale face is rigid, but my eyes are alert, and I press my shoulders down and back, looping a stray hair behind my ear. I pinch my cheeks and take in a deep breath. The men upstairs need me. I am capable.

The clean uniform brings a sense of renewal and confidence. I'm where I should be, where I need to be, and where I will make a difference.

I will survive today, and there will be a new day tomorrow.

25

DECEMBER 1941

SEVEN DAYS HAVE PASSED since watching the last peaceful sunrise and welcoming a new day with hope and joy. The beauty of this tropical paradise is now quiet, dismal, and tattered. Six days have come and gone since President Roosevelt declared America to be at war. Since then, I've had little time to consider the meaning of his words, but in the moments when I'm alone with my thoughts, I compare it to children fighting over wooden blocks and how easy it is to split up the toys and give each child equal parts. Although war could never be as simple as trading a few blocks, I can't understand why ruining so many innocent lives is the answer either.

Then I ponder the other side of the story—a story where we, as Americans, have no choice but to fight for what we believe is right and just. Men and women are stepping forward, potentially giving up their lives to fight for our country. The enemy unfairly attacked, killed, and shattered us. I want to believe we aren't in this battle merely to retaliate, but I suppose a response is what the Japanese requested, and a war is the only way.

I've heard the radio reports and seen the streets outside of the base. Men are standing in lines, waiting to enlist, and women are volunteering to cover duties the men will leave behind. Americans are ready to take back what they have stolen from us.

I've wondered what Mom would think at this moment. Would

she be pro war or against it? Or would she be somewhere in the middle, fighting for a unique solution no one is considering? Her goal was to save people and if our people are going abroad to fight, the ones saving them need to follow in their footsteps.

All along I thought I had to decide between taking a nursing position on the East Coast or the West Coast, but there is a third option, and it's going against Dad's wishes. My safety and well-being will be in jeopardy but if I have a purpose in life, like Mom said, I no longer see the other two career opportunities fulfilling the role I believe I can handle.

The Red Cross has mounted flyers to recruit our nation on every free inch of space. I have never seen so many people in the streets this early in the morning, waiting to sign their names away to Uncle Sam. A sharp red poster catches my eye on the window of a closed hair salon.

The image of a beautiful woman decked in army greens and decorated with gold insignias. Her bright eyes are bigger than the sky, as if she's enough to take on the world, one wound at a time.

YOU ARE NEEDED NOW
JOIN THE
ARMY NURSE CORPS

It's as if she's speaking directly to me, calling me to join her in this fight we will not concede. The fine print on the bottom of the notice states to visit the local Red Cross station to apply.

The Red Cross moved into a vacant space down the street, and there has been a line of people in front of the location since last Monday. Dad will not agree with my decision, but I can't justify not doing more. I have the training and the registered nurse license needed, and I will be twenty-one in just two weeks. I'm unmarried and a citizen of this country. This is my obligation and my right.

Images of Everett and I running along the shore at the beach flash through my mind. The happy days, the star-filled nights, the sensation of his arms around me, the way he looks in my eyes have felt like nothing I ever imagined feeling. I will always treasure and hold on to those memories, and I pray there will be more because he is my one, but I can't let love alter what I must do.

The walk down the sidewalk feels longer than the true distance as I keep my sights set toward the mountain tops on the horizon. My pulse races, but not with fear. The decision for my future is unsettling, but clear. I no longer have only two options to choose from. I set the third path to the side until now. Although the troublesome feeling of going against the wishes of my loved ones is a struggle and is weighing heavily on me, it's what is best. I have a skill the country desperately needs, and it's difficult to avoid the pleas for help on every street corner.

The magnetic pull toward my future is unbreakable until I approach the door covered with informative Red Cross posters. I pause and place the back of my hand against my mouth, taking a moment to think this through once more.

I'm capable.

I meet the requirements and don't have a future that's etched in stone.

With a deep breath held within my lungs, I reach for the door and step inside. One other woman is here at this hour and she's holding a packet of papers, heading for the door.

"May I help you?" a middle-aged woman dressed in a white uniform with a navy-blue cape and a red cross patch sewn above her left breast asks. Her hair is dark and pinned up in perfect curls, covered by a crisp white cap with a matching embroidered red cross to the one on her chest. Her makeup is pristine, and she looks like the women on the Red Cross posters in town.

"Good morning, yes, I would like to enlist in the Army Nurse Corps."

The nurse smiles, her vivid, cardinal-red lipstick is a stark contrast against her brilliantly white teeth. "Wonderful, I assume you are familiar with the requirements to apply?"

"Yes, Ma'am." I reach into my pocketbook, retrieving the paperwork. "I'm two weeks shy of turning twenty-one, but I would like to get the process started."

"Certainly," the nurse says, taking the papers from my hand.

"I have some paperwork you will need to fill out while I enter your information into the database. Do you have questions I can answer before you proceed with this process?"

I smile to match hers. "No, Ma'am, I've grown up here on base. My father is a commander in the Navy, my brothers are both enlisted, and I feel the calling is in my blood, as well." I might have joined the Navy Nurse Corps if the age requirement wasn't twenty-eight, but everything falls into place where needed, right?

"It's helpful to be familiar with military protocol. We are requiring basic training and some course work for new recruits. Some training might be physically vigorous, so I feel it's necessary to warn you for what is ahead."

I wasn't sure what they might involve in training, but I'm not surprised to hear her statements. "Of course, I would expect nothing less." It will be in my best interest to exercise more than I have been.

"Once you are through with your paperwork, I will submit your application to the Army Nurse Corps, and you will probably hear from an officer shortly. Once I submit the paperwork, please understand that the signature on the form you are signing is a commitment and agreement to follow through with your intention to serve."

"Yes, Ma'am, I understand." I place the pen down on the paper and begin filling out the questionnaire.

"This lifestyle can be quite exotic too. You will be able to travel and see parts of the world you never imagined. The Army is truly an opportunity of a lifetime and I'm sure you will be happy with your decision."

I take in her words as I continue to write out my information. To see the world is a dream, but I'm not foolish enough to think that this type of travel will be luxurious. We are amid a war, and there is nothing glorious about this. I am here to put my skills to use and help in any way possible.

Within a few minutes, I complete the paperwork and hand over my lifelong commitment. "Thank you for your time," I offer.

"Thank you for your desire to serve our country," she replies.

Once I step back onto the curb, I feel a sense of fulfillment and relief that I made my decision and there is no turning back. The day looks a little brighter, and the sun feels a little warmer. "Is this what *purpose* feels like?" I whisper to the wind, asking Mom as if she were walking beside me.

On my walk back to the hospital where I will continue volunteering for the time being, thoughts of Everett slip back into my mind—thoughts I tried to block out as I filled out the forms at the Red Cross. Will he still stand by me and respect my decision when I tell him what I've done? Will he feel hurt that I didn't ask his opinion before I signed the papers? More importantly, will we be together in fifty years, sitting on rocking chairs, holding hands on our porch?

Or will I remember this day as one where I ended *us*?

I pass the small diner I often visit for lunch or a Sunday morning brunch occasionally. The place is still fairly empty. Many people are too scared to leave their homes unless necessary. We are all justified to feel that way.

"Lizzie!" I turn toward the sound of my name, finding Audrey and her mother walking out of the diner. I didn't notice her while walking by, so I'm caught off guard to find them staring at me with curious eyes. I can assume they might be curious why I'm down here alone at this time of day.

With an attempt to act casual, I run up to my best friend and wrap my arms around her neck. "I didn't know you were going out for breakfast this morning."

Audrey has been working long hours in one of the field hospitals near the Marine base where she was placed to spend her time rather than in the Naval hospital where she took a nursing position. I step over to her mother next and embrace her tightly. She can't hide the sadness within her eyes, no matter how much makeup she applies. She has looked the same since I first found Audrey this past Tuesday. It was a long couple of days left wondering if she was all right, but luckily, she and her family are fine too. "Mrs. Evans, how are you doing today?" I ask.

"Oh, you know, same as everyone else walking around with a look of hopelessness in their eyes, I suppose." She isn't shy about what she's feeling, and I believe it's best to speak one's mind. A person bottling up their emotions will erupt at some point. There is no simple way to digest the shift in our lives.

"I know the look well," I offer in response. "How is Mr. Evans doing?" I used to refer to him by his ranking, but our families are closer than military neighbors. We're more like family and embrace that feeling.

"I assume much like your dad. He's quiet, angry, restless, and the thoughts spinning in his head are endless."

"Same here, my dad has been pulling some long days and I don't believe he has slept much at all this week."

"Are the twins okay?" Mrs. Evans asks.

"Yes, they've been in and out but also working more hours too."

"You know you are more than welcome to come stay with us while no one is home, right? We have discussed this in the past and you do not need an invitation to walk through our doors, and that goes for any time of day or night."

"I appreciate the offer, Mrs. Evans. Maybe I can make something to bring over for supper one night this week."

Mrs. Evans shoos her white-gloved hand in my direction. "Nonsense, Elizabeth, don't be silly. You can be our guest. You don't need to bring anything."

Audrey is staring at me as if she has a burning question. "Is everything okay?" I ask her.

"Mom, could you give us just a moment?" Audrey asks Mrs. Evans.

Mrs. Evans peers between Audrey and me, then adjusts the tilt of her gray pillbox hat that matches her skirt. She appears suspicious of what we would need to speak about in private, as am I. "Of course." Mrs. Evans tilts her head to the right, peering around us, down the sidewalk. "As a matter of fact, I need to run into the pharmacy at the corner. I'll be just a few minutes. I look forward to seeing you one night this week, dear," she says before walking off toward the corner.

"Goodbye, Mrs. Evans," I call out with a wave.

"What is in your hand?" Audrey asks, grabbing my wrist to flip over.

"Nothing," I say, tugging away from her hold.

"Open your hand, Lizzie." Audrey isn't shy about prying my fingers open from my tight grip, exposing the Red Cross button the nurse handed me in exchange for my paperwork. "Did you donate more blood this morning?"

I stare my friend squarely in the eyes. "No, I did not donate more blood this morning."

Audrey shakes her head with dismay as a fleeting look of pain burns through her eyes. "You didn't ..."

"It's what is best for me and I feel it's my purpose in life."

Audrey releases my hand and gently pinches her fingers around the star dangling from my necklace. "They will kill you over there if you deploy. Why would you do this? You know what is happening in Europe, Elizabeth. You are a smart woman, so why would you be so reckless at a time like this?"

I can't say her words don't hurt me, but I understand her concern for my well-being.

"Audrey, I don't have a say on being a Jewish woman, and the men who died without a chance to fight, here, in our country, didn't have a choice either. It doesn't matter who we are, where we are, or what we are doing. Our lives seem to have a plan, one we may not be aware of yet. Can't you see?"

"No, I can't see. We're lucky to be alive after what has happened this past week. Have you not seen enough? I know I have."

Her question isn't fair because I've seen more than I could have ever imagined witnessing, and I certainly don't wish for more of what we experienced, but all the men standing in a line across the street will depend on us just as we are counting on them.

"These young men are going to need us, Audrey. And if we aren't there, they could die in vain while fighting for the freedom we hold so dearly. I can't sit back and simply hope for the best."

Audrey crosses her arms over her chest and purses her lips with a glimpse of disappointment "This is a foolish decision, Elizabeth. It's just plain foolish. You don't know that you won't be whisked away to one of those horrid camps in Germany if someone finds out you are Jewish."

"You mean, like what they are doing to some innocent Japanese civilians here?" I respond in a lower voice.

"Elizabeth, you know that is a different situation."

"No, it's not. We're afraid of them because of their race, but there is no reason to be fearful of every confined person. It's not right."

"You have lost your mind, Elizabeth. You don't know what you are saying. Maybe your mind got jumbled during those explosions."

"You can't be serious."

"Are you hoping they lock you up in Germany because the Germans are afraid of Jews? They won't stop to wonder if you are a good Jewish person. Just the same as no one is stopping to think that most, if not all, of the Japanese in the camps here are good people. That isn't the way war works. It's a life for a life, and your life would be on the line first."

"We're women too. I guess we have nothing good going for us, do we?"

"How dare you speak that way?" Audrey and I have had our moments arguing over silly topics, but we have never had a fight that has ended with us making each other feel terrible. We love each other like sisters, but I need her to understand where I'm coming from.

"It's true, Audrey. I don't agree with society's views, and if I'm locked up for being a Jewish woman, then I will be a lesson to the world someday. Whatever the case, I need to make a difference somehow—someway, and that is what I'm going to do."

Audrey folds her arms over her chest and grits her jaw tightly. "Have you told Everett or your father yet?"

"No, this was my decision, and mine alone to make."

"You are going to break their hearts, Elizabeth, and we've already been through so much."

There's nothing more to say. It's not my intention to cause anyone I love pain, but I can't allow anyone to stand in my way of what I must do. "I appreciate your honesty."

Audrey lunges forward, wrapping her arms around me, holding me tightly. "I'm so angry at you, Elizabeth Salzberg, but I love you. Don't forget that."

"I love you too. We're going to be okay. We're going to be better than okay."

My promising statement is full of meaningless words. Nothing is truly okay, and there are no guarantees on how anyone's future will turn out with what we are facing.

26

DECEMBER 1941

IF THERE IS one way to everyone's heart in this house, it's meatloaf. Personally, I could go a year without seeing another chopped, formed, brick-shaped glob of beef, but this meal isn't for me, per se. Plus, the meat alone will be a surprise since the commissary has been low on goods due to panic rationing. Meat hasn't been in stock since Wednesday, but I had this package of hamburger sitting in the freezer box so I can save my worry about food for another night.

Dad told James and Lewis to be home by a decent hour for supper tonight because he's concerned the three of them are going to burn out at this rate. The cleanup at Pearl is never ending. I don't see how we'll ever get this base back to the condition it was in. Never mind the battleships. They nearly destroyed all eight, and no one is sure if any are salvageable yet. It's all hands-on deck, but with so many injuries, the burden is heavy on those fortunate enough to have walked away in one piece.

The more I consider their exhaustion, the worse I feel about the news I'm going to be delivering tonight. Not even meatloaf will lessen the impact of my news. I'm not sure how long it takes papers to process through the system or when someone from the Army Nurse Corps will contact me about my application, so I have to get this over with.

With the sun setting at this early hour, headlights are already lighting up the road in front of the house. I must seem like an anxious child, jumping at every sound and sight of a car, waiting for Everett to pull up out front. I asked him to join us for dinner tonight too, but I believe he will be here sooner than the rest of them so I can talk to him privately before they get home. My decision probably won't be as much of a shock to him as my family, but I'm not naïve to Everett's feelings on the matter. He supports my endeavors in every way possible, but his fear of what's occurring in Europe overrides his support for me enlisting. And then there's also the *"us"* part of this—love is hard to fight against.

It's tough going against what everyone else wants, but I'm at a crossroad where I know my feelings must count more than anyone else's. I haven't made this decision lightly. I have wanted to join the Army Nurse Corps for a long time, but I might have let go of the dream after receiving two job offers. Now everything has changed, and I'm doing what I believe is right.

After whipping the mashed potatoes with blunt force for a few minutes too long, I pause to catch my breath and spot a set of headlights parked out front. He didn't pull into the driveway, so it must be Everett. I wipe my hands clean on a dish towel and race to the front door, eager to see the eyes I think about all day.

"What do you have all over you, doll-face?" Everett asks while approaching the storm door.

I glance down at my dress and apron, wondering what he's looking at. "There is nothing on me, silly. Maybe you are hallucinating after another long day."

The moment he walks through the door, I smell the fresh scent of soap and the spice of his aftershave. He's wearing an aquamarine floral-print aloha shirt. The vanity of living in Hawaii suits him well. The bright colors against his bronze tan make him even more appealing than when he's dressed in all neutral colors. "You don't think you have anything on you?" he continues, teasing me with a coy smirk.

"How in the world do you have this much energy for horseplay at this hour of the day?"

Everett scoops his arm around my back and pulls my waist in against his. His eyes burn into mine for a long breathless second, but then his free hand reaches for my face and he sweeps his thumb across the width of my left cheek. "Hmm." He inspects his finger, then dips it into his mouth. "Just as I thought. Mashed potatoes."

I pull away from his hold and swat at his arm. "Why, I've never—"

"Never, what, doll-face? Gotten potatoes on your face? We've all been there."

"All these long hours have stolen the gentleman right out of you, Lieutenant Anderson."

"Aw, come on, baby, you can't take a little teasing? That isn't like you. Is everything all right?" Everett reaches for me once more and pulls me back into his embrace. "Yeah, something isn't right. I can see it in your eyes. They aren't twinkling like they normally do. You got yourself in trouble today, didn't you?" I suppose I can't say Everett doesn't notice every single detail about me.

"Am I that obvious?" I question.

Everett's smile fades and he glides the back of his hand along the side of my face. "What's wrong, Lizzie?"

"Nothing is wrong." I try to swallow the lump in my throat, but the way he's looking at me, it makes my body weak. "I—I just decided on something today and acted on it before anyone would have the chance to talk me out of it."

Everett closes his eyes, his dark lashes sweep across his high cheekbones, and he holds his palm up to the side of his face. "You enlisted." He isn't asking. He knows.

"Everett, I know it's not what you or anyone wants for me, but you must understand, it's my calling and I can't ignore the thoughts reeling through my head. I am positive I am cut out to be a part of the Army Nurse Corps. You can't argue. You just can't. We both know it's only a matter of time before you receive orders for a deployment, and I refuse to sit here like a lady and wait for all the blood, sweat and tears to pass before our nation becomes safe again. I can't imagine the helpless feeling of not being where I'm needed—wherever that may be."

"I understand, Lizzie. Believe me, I get it. I will not stand in your way or make you think your decision isn't right. Over the past week, you have proven your strength, courage, and determination in a way that I've never seen before. I see why you feel like this is your direction. I feel the same way about my own."

I take Everett's hands within mine. "You know, I don't want you to think the thought of us, you and me, our future hasn't crossed my mind, but we're going to have all the time in the world for that after the war ends. I'm sure my decision would have been harder if you were a civilian. The thought of leaving you behind breaks my heart into millions of pieces, but neither of us will leave the other behind. We both have duties to fulfill before we can reach a point where there are no obstacles between us."

Everett pulls in a long inhale. "Everything you said is accurate, Lizzie. It's going to be hard not worrying about you, though."

I place my hand on his chest and stare up into his eyes. "We can't think that way. If this world has a plan for us, which I believe in my heart, it does, then we will be together after this is over. We have to have faith in fate. Don't you believe everything happens for a reason?"

"What does fate think about all the tomorrows and yesterday's?" Everett asks, his heart pounding beneath my hand.

"Fate outweighs the days, weeks, and months—it outweighs time. Fate is where we end up when we end up there. Knowing you will be there is all the determination I need to keep my focus where it should be. It will get me through the long days, nights, and months. It will carry me through until we win this battle."

Another set of headlights flashes against the living room window. "Is that your father?"

"Probably."

"You haven't told him yet, have you?"

I drop my gaze down between our feet. "I was hoping you might be next to me when I do."

Everett lifts his hand to cover his eyes for a moment. "I thought you said we were both going to survive this, Lizzie? I'm going to be lucky if I make it out of this house alive tonight."

"There are worse ways to go, right?"

"You know, you're right. Everything you have said over the last ten minutes couldn't be further from the truth because I honestly feel deep down in my heart that you, Elizabeth Salzberg, will probably be the death of me." A soft chuckle emits from his mouth before I press up on my toes to steal a quick kiss before Dad walks into the house.

The moment the door opens, Everett clicks his heels together and tosses his hand up to salute Dad.

"Everett, I didn't know you'd be joining us tonight. Put your hand down, son. You're off duty." Dad greets him, before me, his daughter, but I'd prefer that over the trying months of wishing Dad would accept Everett as my boyfriend rather than Mr. Hollywood, as he referred to him until recently.

Dad turns around and kisses me on the forehead. His eyebrow rises with skepticism as he glances at my face but doesn't pursue a line of questioning for the time being. "I'm going to rinse off and change out of uniform. I'll be ready for supper shortly. Your brothers are due home any moment now too," Dad says before heading down toward his bedroom.

"It seems my father has taken a liking to you," I say, pinching Everett's chin. With a pivot of my heels, I return to the kitchen to check on the simmering candied carrots.

"The house smells like a slice of heaven, Lizzie. Do I smell meatloaf?" Everett questions, reaching for the metal handle of the oven.

I swat at his hand with the dish towel. Don't touch. I want to keep the steam inside. "But, yes, meatloaf—"

"Whipped potatoes," he continues with a wink.

"And candied-carrots," I finish.

"You outdid yourself tonight. How did you get all this done after volunteering at the hospital all day?"

I point my potholder at him. "Never question a woman's ability to perform magic."

Everett holds his hands up in defense. "Yes, Ma'am. Well, I'm thankful for the kind invitation to join you all for a showdown tonight, and the deliciously smelling meatloaf too."

The nerves in my belly fizzle again after nearly forgetting my intentions of winning my family over with their favorite meal. Everett uses the free time to inspect the framed portraits hanging on the wall between the kitchen and family room. They have been hanging in the same spot since I was a child. Mom loved family portraits, even though James and Lewis often fooled with her about hanging up photographs of the people she sees more than anyone else in the world. *Why look at a picture when you can look directly at us in living form?*

"Someday, these portraits will be important to you. They represent a moment in time that you will long for again. You may not appreciate these framed beauties now, but there will come a day when they will be the reason you smile first thing in the morning," she said often.

"Your hair was so light when you were younger, and those freckles," Everett calls over.

"My mom was a natural blonde, and I got those good genes, I guess."

"Where did your freckles go? They don't just disappear," he continues.

"Everett, must I explain this to you again? Never question a woman's ability to perform magic." Thank goodness for cosmetics because my freckles make me look like a child.

"You look just like her, you know. She was beautiful."

"Thank you. I get that a lot."

I finish setting up the table just as James and Lewis walk through the door. I didn't even notice their headlights flash by.

"Anderson, how are you hanging in there this week? Are they working you to the bone on the airfield too?"

"Yes, it's been quite the mess to clean up, but I doubt it is comparable to what you've had to handle at the piers."

"Go clean up and change. Supper is just about ready," I tell the boys.

"Oh, hey there, sis," James says with a snicker. "How was *your* day today?"

Everett, in a not-so-inconspicuous manner, turns away from the conversation to continue gazing at the wall of portraits. The silence is full of narrowing eyes set on me from both James and Lewis.

"Elizabeth, what did you do today other than volunteer and make something for supper that smells like my favorite meal?"

"I worked, cooked, and cleaned. Why, what else is there for a woman to do?"

"I will ignore the sarcasm and take a hint. We'll be ready for supper in a couple minutes," Lewis says.

James approaches Everett and slaps his hand down on his shoulder. "Check out Elizabeth without her front teeth. It took forever for them to grow back in and she had the cutest little lisp for years after." I choose to roll my eyes when James tries to poke fun at me. I learned a long time ago that jabbing back in a teasing contest often leads to family feuds, so I do what I usually do, and ignore James's attempts to antagonize me

"We all go through that awkward phase," Everett responds.

"Oh, come on, there's no way you had awkward years," Lewis says while walking down the hall toward his bedroom.

"Lucky for me, I don't have those mortifying photographs here with me," Everett mutters. "I left those beauties for my dad to enjoy."

"Well, darn," I reply. "I would love to see those."

Dad returns to the dinette table, wearing an oddly similar shirt to the one Everett has on. "I don't remember the last time I've worn one of these babies. I almost forgot what it feels like to wear color," Dad says.

"Dad, where did you even find that shirt? That must be from 1930."

"I've had it in my closet waiting for a reason to wear it again." Tonight, is hardly a reason to wear an aloha shirt in this house, but if it lifts his mood even slightly, I'll be thankful. The guilt is heavy, and I know I'm about to ruin his night. I tried to avoid the thought of telling Dad about my decision, but I must come clean and stay strong.

James and Lewis join us in their usual white t-shirts and slacks. "Hey Anderson, did you catch the line of new recruits filling the street today?" James asks.

"Please show our guest a little respect," Dad snaps at James. "He is a lieutenant. You know better."

Lewis walks in on the conversation and we're all awkwardly staring at each other. Dad wasn't exactly a part of our "family" supper outings when James and Lewis wanted to get to know

Everett. The three of them formed a nice friendship and had dropped the addressing of rank names several months ago.

"With all due respect, Sir, I don't mind when I'm in your house. It's nice to leave work at work sometimes, as I'm sure you understand."

"Of course, son. I wanted to make sure you didn't feel disrespected."

"No at all," Everett says with a dip of his head.

"Please, everyone sit down before the loaf gets cold."

"How were you able to find meat anywhere this week?" Lewis asks.

"It's the last of what we have. I had it in the freezer. I'll drive off base next week to see if other grocery stores have a better supply."

Moments after everyone settles down at the table and helps themselves to each dish, Dad takes a swig of wine and gently places the glass down, keeping his gaze set on the red liquid sloshing around. "Elizabeth, the only time you make meatloaf is when you want to cheer us up, or if you have something you need to tell us that will probably cause a storm of anger. I'm eager to hear which of these situations is your motivation this evening," Dad says.

Everett chokes on the mouthful of wine he has in his mouth and clears his throat. "You see, Elizabeth, here, doesn't care for meatloaf all that much, but she knows we enjoy the meal. So, when she makes this dish, it's easy to tell there's something hiding behind the mouthwatering taste she's distracting us with," James adds.

It is truly difficult living in a house full of men who have far too much training in intelligence. I can never hide much of anything from them, which is why I'm nearly positive Dad had a blind eye to my rendezvous with Everett throughout the summer. Surely, he knew something was going on, but decided not to let on until that day at the air show.

"We've all had a tough week, and I thought it might be nice to enjoy your favorite meal tonight," I say, sounding sheepish compared to the way I intended to sound.

"I know what this is about," Lewis says. "You finally decided which job you're going to take, didn't you?" Lewis and I have had many conversations on the topic over the last couple months. Neither position would take me on until after the new year, so time has been ticking by slowly as I have weighed each option over and over, not able to decide until this week.

"As a matter of fact, yes, I have made a decision, and that is what I want to share with you all tonight." From the corner of my eye, I watch Everett polish off the wine from his glass.

"Clearly, you've shared the news with Everett already," Dad says before clearing his throat and dabbing his napkin across his lips. "Well, let's hear it then."

I've been clutching my napkin between my fist for the last minute of this conversation and I notice the whites of my knuckles glowing from beneath the table. I release the napkin and fold my hands together, preparing myself for the wrath I expect.

"Well, I decided, without influence, to apply for the Army Nurse Corps today." I'm not sure whose fork hits the fine china first, but a succession of loud clinks pierces my ears.

"You all realize you will probably deploy soon, correct?" Dad asks with despair in his eyes.

"Yes, Elizabeth, and the last thing we need is to worry about you being deployed. Why would you do this after everything we talked about?" Lewis asks.

"For the record, before anyone else says another word, Everett just found out moments before you got home. He was not aware of my decision when I made it. None of you agree with what I feel is important for my life. I did what I needed to do."

"Will you excuse me for a moment?" Dad asks. The wooden legs from his chair scrape against the floor just before he walks directly out the front door.

James has resumed eating the meatloaf, keeping his eyes fixed on the plate of food. Everett reaches beneath the table for my hand and collapses his fingers between mine. "You should go talk to him," he suggests.

I place my napkin down on my chair as I stand up and follow Dad's path out the front door. He has a cigarette pinched between his lips and he's staring up at the stars. "Last week wasn't enough for you?" he asks.

"On the contrary, last week proved to me that I'm cut from the same cloth as you, James, and Lewis. I helped so many men over the last week, and though it was extremely challenging to maintain my composure while watching so much death and destruction, I felt like I was there in that place because it was my calling. If we're going to war, our men are going to need the same care overseas as they did here."

"I understand what it feels like to follow this 'calling' you are referring too. However, this war will not end anytime soon, Elizabeth, and what you witnessed here this past week could be much worse overseas. You do not know where you might end up. So many countries are a part of this, and we are allies to half of them. I lived through the first World War, Elizabeth. It was a time no one should have to live through twice, but here we are, moving forward just over twenty years later."

"I'm not part of the cause, Dad. I want to be a piece of the solution. My intentions are not to join in a battle. I want to help those who are fighting on behalf of our country and the allies. It's my right to feel this way."

"Your mother didn't want this for you. She was adamant about you staying out of the military."

"Mom stood up for what was moral, and she fought for changes and women's empowerment. Women's rights are what she supported, Dad, and this is my right."

"I'm at a loss for words, Elizabeth. I can't tell you I'm disappointed in you because frankly, I'm quite proud, but you are my daughter, and I am terrified for your well-being." Dad finally turns to look at me, pulling the cigarette from his lips. "There's not much else I can say."

"I understand," I respond, pressing up on my toes to kiss his cheek. "Supper is getting cold."

I was expecting to hear some shouting, more glare radiating from his eyes, but there is only sadness written across his face. It's the way I have felt any time he has had to deploy or take part in a dangerous mission. I have felt that way about Lewis and James several times too. On top of that, I dealt with losing Mom. No one else has focused on the anguish I have lived with over the years, and if they have, they were good at hiding it. "Is Dad calling

General Marshall tomorrow to pull your application?" James asks, holding his glass of wine in hand.

"No, Dad is learning how to accept that I'm a grown woman and he will move on just like we've all had to."

Everett is pale, his knee is bouncing, and he hasn't touched his food since I left. "Your food is going to get cold. Please eat."

Everett looks up at me, then casts his glance toward the front door. "Elizabeth, I need to show your father some respect still. I'm in his house."

I take my seat and whip my napkin across my lap and fold my hands down on top of the table. "Fine. We can all eat cold food, except for James."

James gives me a look like I've insulted him. It wasn't my intention, but it's hard to be kind when there is such a lack of support within this family. Dad re-enters the house, bringing in a waft of smoke behind him. He doesn't smoke often, only when he is feeling anxious. He has been smoking like a chimney over the past week, but it's understandable.

"Please, eat your supper before it gets cold. Elizabeth was kind enough to prepare it for us all," Dad says. I'm a bit surprised to hear his calm tone and change of attitude, but I don't question it. Maybe I said the words he needed to hear.

"Yes, please eat," I repeat.

"So, Everett, I've been told your team has made some good headway with repairs this week. It was some much-needed relief to hear of your progress."

I can hear the trouble Everett has swallowing the bite of food in his mouth. "Yes, Sir, we made a good dent, but we still have a way to go."

"We'll get there. I have faith," Dad says, skating his gaze toward me. "Right, Elizabeth? That's what your mother always said to us: 'Faith is belief, and one should hold on to it dearly.'"

I'm not sure if Dad's words should make me rethink my decision or if he is finally seeing the world through my eyes.

"I couldn't agree more," Everett says.

About a month has passed since the attack on Pearl. Life as we once knew it has yet to return to any sort of normalcy. I'm not sure it ever will ever feel quite the same.

I have been temporarily assisting at the Naval hospital, waiting on initial orders from the Army Nurse Corps. The enlisted men are all still working never-ending days to repair and replace the abundance of damage. I have been wondering if they might be luckier than the rest of us on base with so much work to focus on. The busier we are, the less time there is to think about what is happening to the world.

Each day, I take a bagged lunch to the shaded area down the street to relieve my head of the commotion inside the hospital. Unfortunately, I can't escape the noises that haunt me the most because they live within my mind. If I could plug my ears to make the explosions and cries stop, I would, but I'd still see the horrific images playing before my eyes. There is nowhere to look without a reminder of the attack.

Even after a month, the shrapnel is still in piles within the grass, beneath the curbs, and even on roofs. The worst visual is watching mothers and children walk by with gas masks dangling from their hands. The military has issued all of us protective gear in case there is another air raid or poison gas attack. To witness a drill is like taking a blow to the stomach, and it makes me question how life can have so little meaning.

The military oversees everything in the state of Hawaii. Our freedom that we have enjoyed feels like a distant memory, and though it's for our protection, many of us silently feel like prisoners in the place we call home. I want to wake up and find this all to have been a nightmare, but when I open my eyes each morning, I realize that the time I spend asleep is my only escape.

Saturdays are like every other day of the week now, but we all sleep in for an extra hour in the morning. Today might be an exception, however, because Dad is having an indiscreet conversation on the telephone. It's rare to hear him speaking so loudly to anyone, never mind this early in the day. My silk French robe, a hand-me-down from Mom that Dad brought her after returning from Europe during the first World War, is hanging over the upholstered armchair within reach. I wrap myself up snuggly, protecting my warm skin from the mild draft whirling around. Once my feet are snug within my house slippers, I tip-toe down the hallway to listen in on the conversation Dad is doing little to hide.

"Yes, Captain, I agree and understand. Of course, the timing isn't favorable for either of us. However, I agree Lieutenant Anderson is the best candidate for this position. I will meet with the colonel today to discuss this transition."

Silence bears its heaviness as I wait to hear what Dad says next. "We saw the paratrooper demonstration a couple months ago. It was a phenomenal demonstration, Captain. In fact, I was watching along with Lieutenant Anderson. The display had him quite enamored, in fact. I'm sure Georgia will suit him well too."

My mouth falls ajar, baffled by the discussion. Of all the men on base, I can't understand why Everett would be a topic of conversation with any captain. I know we both understood the probability of deployments, but he's going to be moved, and I can't help but wonder if Dad has something to do with this, or why he would do such a thing.

I flee from the door as the phone call ends with the sound of the receiver clapping with a ding against receiver. With silent movements, I close myself into my bedroom, pondering how I can

warn Everett before the colonel approaches him. I shouldn't have
been eavesdropping and I have no right interfering, but this feels
like the beginning to a very long uphill road ahead—one he might
want a say in. Though I'm not ignorant to the way orders come in,
this situation feels unusual.

With eagerness rushing through my body, I find fresh clothes
and smooth out the bed-worn imperfections in my hair. I look
simply exhausted, but there isn't a person living within a ten-mile
radius who doesn't appear as weary.

In less than ten minutes, I'm out of the house, lifting the
kickstand from my bicycle. I spot Audrey outside, picking weeds
from their front garden. I must be quick with my hello. There still
seems to be a bit of tension between us, but I can say the same
with my family as well. No one understands my decision for
enlisting, and we have all agreed to disagree.

I slowly crawl to a stop in front of her driveway, hearing the
squeal of my brakes, which reminds me to grease the gears later
this afternoon.

"Where are you off so early this morning?" Audrey calls out,
her hand cupped over her eyes to shield away the sun.

"Oh, I have to talk to Everett before he reports to duty this
morning. It's nothing important."

"You have the afternoon free, don't you?"

It's the first Saturday I have had any free time over the last
month. "I do. How about yourself?"

"Surprisingly, yes, I do too. I was wondering if you would like
to come over for some tea today?"

"I'd like that, yes. What time shall we say?"

"How about a bit after noon?"

"I'll be here," I confirm.

"Wonderful, ride safely," she calls out with a wave.

I feel like I just had a conversation with an old acquaintance,
not my best friend. For as long as Audrey and I have been friends,
there has never been an awkward pause or a moment to wonder if
her thoughts match the words she's speaking. It feels awful to
think something has come between us. I can only hope a little
alone time with some tea and gossip can patch up whatever is
wrong with our friendship today.

My light sweater billows in the wind as I pedal down through town. The chilly draft I felt earlier this morning is more like a cool breeze along the shore. It must be cooler than sixty degrees, which isn't typical for Hawaii.

I run my fingers through my hair and pull my tube of lipstick from my dress pocket to refresh the color on my lips. With little makeup on, the least I can do is have a bright hue somewhere on my face to brighten it when greeting Everett this early in the morning.

My fist beating against his door doesn't cause any alarm or rattle from within his barrack. "Everett, it's Lizzie," I announce through the door. After a long second, I hear the squeal from the rusty springs in his mattress. He must have been asleep still. I glance down at my wristwatch, finding the time to be only seven in the morning. I should have waited a little longer before waking him on the one day he can sleep in but knowing Everett he would only leave enough time to wake up, shower and dress before needing to report to duty.

The metal bolt lock releases and he opens the door a few inches, enough for the sun to cast a burning glow against his minty eyes. He's only dressed in his skivvies, his hair is in a tousled mess, and by the look written within the angle of his eyebrows, he appears perplexed about my reason for being here when we have plans tonight. "Is everything all right, doll-face?"

"I'm not sure," I say, trying to be honest. While the idea of Everett leaving is terrible, I need to know what his thoughts are before telling him how I truly feel.

He reaches outside for my elbow and pulls me into his room, closing then bolting the door shut. For someone who wears a uniform during most of his waking hours, he still has the tan of a Hawaiian god. He says he tans easily, but sometimes I wonder if those boys take breaks and sit out on the tarmacs to get a little sun in the middle of the day. "I would have rather woken up next to you than to the sound of your fist against the door," he says, grabbing a white t-shirt from the neatly stacked pile of laundered undergarments on his bureau.

"You know weekdays are the only times I can get away without the interrogation from my father."

"You're a grown woman, Lizzie. We shouldn't need to sneak around anymore. Your father wasn't born yesterday. I'm sure he knows what an adult relationship entails." Everything Everett is saying is true, but until I move out of that house, I'm doing what I can to keep the peace.

"If I had my way, I would be here every night."

"If I had my way, we'd run away and get married before either of us gets sent away," he says.

His words feel like tiny knives plunging into my heart. I didn't see myself as the type to be in a rush to get married. I wasn't the type. I'm still not because I wouldn't dream of doing such a thing while we're on the brink of whatever happens next in this war. But the thought plays out like a fairytale in my head during the nights I'm not here with him. "I wouldn't be able to be in the Army Nurse Corps," I remind him.

"I know, and while I'd like to say that would be the ideal reason to go get married right now, I wouldn't ask that of you."

"That's the reason I love you, Everett Anderson. A piece of gold and a sheet of paper telling me what I already know doesn't make a difference in what the future holds for us. I'm yours. That will never change."

"Well, I'm yours, so don't forget that when some soldier is trying to get your attention with their baby blues, begging you to nurse them back to health."

"That look doesn't work on me, Mr. Anderson. You should know better."

"I'm just fooling with you." Everett presses his hands against the sides of my shoulders and pulls me in to interrupt our conversation with a kiss that steals every last breath from my lungs, leaving me weak and without the motivation to speak. The warmth of his skin against my hands is a feeling I will keep with me whenever we are apart. My arms fit perfectly against the sides of his back muscles. I press my cheek to his chest, closing my eyes to keep the moment going for as long as I can before spoiling everything with the news I overheard. "You drive me wild, Lizzie, you know that?"

I snicker quietly and take a step back to allow him to pull his shirt over his head. "I'm afraid I overheard a conversation this morning that I shouldn't have."

Everett straightens his white shirt and crosses his arms over his chest. "What do you mean?"

"I woke up to the sound of a conversation coming from the dining room. My father was on the phone with a Captain, but I'm not sure which one. They were discussing orders and mentioned your name as the most suitable candidate for the position in Georgia. Apparently, my father is due to talk to your colonel today."

Everett's brows rise then fall, his mouth parts, and he takes a couple of steps backward to sit on the edge of his bed. "Georgia. Fort Benning is in Georgia. That's where the paratroopers train." I realize now is not the time to remind Everett about his decision to remain a pilot rather than the man jumping out of a plane, but he may not have a say, I suppose. "Did your dad recommend me?"

I shrug my shoulders and clasp my hands together, feeling guilty for only reporting the part of the conversation I heard. "It was hard to tell from the time I listened in. It sounded as if they had already mentioned your name and my father agreed you are the best candidate for the position."

Everett lifts his stare, focusing on my eyes as shock fades from his tense shoulders. "I don't know what to say, Lizzie."

"Is this something you want?" I ask. I don't think it matters, but if he must go, I'd prefer to know he doesn't hate the idea.

Everett stands up from his bed and locks his hands on his hips. "You're asking me an impossible question. Yes, I want to work with the paratroopers. Hell, it's the reason I enlisted, but you've made all that change, and I don't mean that in a bad way. I'd jump off a cliff if it meant having more time with you for a little longer, but we both know that wouldn't change a thing and we are holding our breath daily, waiting for your orders to come in."

"Everett, you are going to be jumping from planes because someone tells you to," I argue, "but that isn't the point. You're right. We both knew what we were doing when we enlisted, and we can't have regrets." *Just heartache.*

"Did he say when this would happen?"

I shake my head. "No, but it's fair to assume things will move along quickly. Act surprised when your colonel approaches you with this information, okay?"

"Of course. That goes without saying, sweetheart."

Everett takes a moment to peer out of his one window, overlooking another barrack building. "We're facing the inevitable and biding our time before one of us has to leave. I can't lie to you and tell you this isn't what I want. In fact, this is beyond any opportunity I could have hoped for in the Air Corps. But, doll, one thing has nothing to do with the other. I want to take you with me."

The thought passes through my mind, an idea I hadn't considered in the last hour. "How would that work? We aren't married, and we couldn't live in the barracks together?"

"I have money, Lizzie. We could get a little place off base."

I must have stars floating above my head at the mere idea of playing house with Everett, but it's only a matter of time before reality kicks in to remind me that at any moment I could receive orders to move anywhere within this country to train. The odds of ending up at Fort Benning are as unlikely as one of us not deploying within the next few months. For the moment, though, and for the sake of his sweet offer, I jump into his arms, lock my legs around his waist, and slap my hands against his cheeks. "That sounds like a dream come true."

"Under one condition, though," he says, pulling his head back to capture my full attention.

"What's that?" I ask, feeling the muscles in my cheeks tighten against my smile.

"Pretend like this is an actual possibility until we find out it's not."

CURRENT DAY - OCTOBER 2018

"Oh, my goodness, Daniel, were you here all day?" The sweet voice is like a melody to my ears, and her face, it's one I never forget no matter how bad a day might be. I study her as she walks gracefully in a shiny pair of black leather stilettos, matched perfectly with her tailored three-piece suit. My granddaughter has the word success written in her eyes. Her confidence plays a fine line between playful and serious, but no one could mistake her look for anger. She speaks softly like her grandfather but owns her contrasting freckles that stand out against her sun-bleached hair. Of course, it's rare to see Makena with her hair down since she believes in keeping her face free from distraction, but when she lets it down, the ringlets I used to coil around my fingers still dangle halfway down her back. It's hard to recall when she transitioned from a giggly little girl to this poised, elegant woman who appears to own the world. I still see the pink cheeks and gaps in her teeth, wet lashes, and crooked pigtails as she ran through the wind on the beach every afternoon until the sun stole every bit of her energy.

"Gran, you sound like you're losing your voice. Are you feeling okay?" Makena asks.

"I'm not losing my voice, sweetheart. I've been helping this nice young man with his research today." I glance down at his notepad, finding it as blank as it was when he arrived this morning.

"Nice young man, huh?" Makena responds with a smirk. "I suppose he is what you say. In fact, I thought so just a year ago when we got married right on that beach down there."

I take in Makena's words, trying to smile in response, but wishing I could recall a word of what she's talking about. She's married to this man. I don't recall.

"Dan, you haven't taken notes," Makena points out with a chuckle.

"I have some notes in the car. I jotted them down while she napped earlier. She painted such vivid pictures; I didn't want to miss anything while looking down at my notebook." I readjust my posture, realizing I haven't moved from this seat since we ate lunch a couple of hours ago. It's time to stretch my legs. Keiki typically reminds me, but I assume she didn't want to interrupt my storytelling.

Makena wraps her hands around my elbow and tugs as I push myself up to my feet. "I remember helping people up like this," I tell my granddaughter. "Now I'm the one who can't stand up without a good heave-ho."

"Oh, Gran," Makena sighs. She keeps her hands nearby and ready in case I stumble like a toddler taking her first steps, but I'm not going far. It's the time of day when the cumulus clouds roll through, their shapes and buoyancy mimic the appearance of a hand-drawn cartoon with unique curves and shading. I once thought clouds looked the same no matter where a person might be in the world, but it wasn't until I began traveling that I noticed how different a cloud looks depending on the weather, elevation, and environment. If there was a contest on which location has the most beautiful clouds, this island would win without a close race.

Makena's hand strokes my upper back as I lean my elbows down on the ledge of the balcony. "That's a horse, without a doubt," she says, pointing at the cloud I was just studying.

"A Clydesdale, to be specific," I counter.

The muffled sound of a bee buzzing pulls my attention away from the horizon in search of the source, but when I glance in

Makena's direction, the pulsating sound halts as she holds her telephone up to her ear.

"Hi," she answers. "What's up?" Makena lifts her gaze from her shoes and finds her reflection in my eyes. "Yes, I'm here. She's great."

Is it me she's speaking about?

"Sure, hold on." Makena reaches her telephone over to me, waiting for me to take it from her hand. I always hate fiddling around with this new technology the kids carry around. It hardly fits in my hand, and I feel like I might drop it. Surely it would shatter into a million pieces if that were to happen. As relentless as Makena is, she holds the telephone up for me until I concede and take the shiny device from her hand, holding it up to my ear.

"Gran, turn it around; it's facing the wrong way." I must look ridiculous, but a true telephone doesn't offer the option of mistakenly holding the receiver incorrectly. With both hands, I turn the piece of glass carefully until it's flipped around.

"Hello?"

"Mom, what have you been up to all day? I've called a few times, but Keiki said you've been busy outside talking Daniel's ear off. Is everything okay?"

I continue holding the phone within both of my hands as I pivot my stance to face the water rather than Makena. "Yes, I've been talking to Daniel for the last few hours. There's no need to worry."

"You don't sound right, Mom."

I close my eyes, focusing on his voice. "I just said there's nothing to worry about," I repeat.

"Okay, well Julia and I will be over soon."

"Well, hold on a moment. I'm not sure Keiki is preparing enough food for all of us tonight. I must speak with her first."

"Mom, I've already spoken to Keiki several times today. Everything is all set."

"What's the occasion for supper on a weeknight?"

"It's Friday night. Leah and Cliff will be over too."

Rather than say goodbye to the man calling me his mother, I hand the phone back to Makena, waiting until it's safe within her grip before I let go. I return my gaze out toward the sea and clouds. "Daniel, did I tell you about my time on the East Coast yet?"

The patio chair scrapes against the terse texture of the flooring as Daniel makes his way to my side. Makena finishes her phone call on the other side of the terrace.

"So, you went with Everett to Georgia?" Daniel asks.

"You know, there's a saying my mother always recited to me and it made little sense until I experienced the meaning."

"What was the saying?" Daniel presses.

I smile and press my lips together. "She would tell me to stop planning out my tomorrows because: 'passionately prepared plans predictably perish.' I wish I had listened to her that one time."

I'M ACTING FOOLISH, walking my bicycle around with this giddy smile on my face. I've had to raise my gloved hand to my face every time a person has passed me on the street. It still doesn't feel right to be cheerful around here, and truthfully, there is little reason to smile unless someone can understand the lifetime of happiness I'm imagining in my mind. It is difficult to block out the debris or pass by the memorials left from vigils along the curb. I stop for a moment and offer a prayer for the lost ones.

This feeling of love is splendid, but I believe I have been avoiding the idea entirely because Mom always said nothing else matters when a woman is dizzy and in love and it's her biggest weakness. She didn't intend for her words to detract me from finding a husband and having a family someday, but to make sure I make my dreams and goals a priority rather than settling for something less than I deserve.

The idea of dating seemed like more trouble than it was worth, mostly because of Dad, but I always enjoyed the attention I would get when out with the girls on a weekend night. It's fun to play hard to get. Or it was. Even though times are different now, I don't miss those nights of teasing boys and leaving them winded, clutching their chest. It was all just a game. I doubt I broke any hearts.

What Everett and I have between us is real. I can feel it deep in my core, and through every bone of my being. It's so intense and distracting that my smile has lasted at least twenty minutes without thinking about my call-to-service: the where, when, and how it will happen. It could be months before I receive orders. At least that is what I heard. I expected to receive the call within days after enlisting, but I haven't heard a peep. So, for now, I will focus on today rather than tomorrow, as I promised to always do. And today, I want to move to Georgia with Everett whenever he must go. Perhaps Georgia could be a place where I am training, too. I could put in a request. Since I haven't received orders yet, they may take my petition into consideration.

My mind is clearly running twenty miles faster than my legs, but a girl can dream, and there's nothing wrong with that. As the jumbled-up thoughts clear out of my brain, a beautiful mahogany coffee table pulls my attention to the window of a home decorating store. I could pick out the decor for our new home. Everett isn't particular around little details like colors, fabrics, or wood types. I can imagine he would follow me around a store with his hands clasped behind his back, stopping short before my heels at every piece of furniture I'd want to examine.

I lean my bicycle against the brick edifice of the row of storefronts, then lift my sunglasses up and settle them on the crown of my head. I'm overcome with a sense of eagerness to slip inside the store that has small living room and bedroom displays set up in a row along the long wall.

"Good morning, Miss. Can I help you with something today?" The store clerk, an older gentleman, who looks like he might have served in the military at a younger age by the way he walks, approaches me at the first display. His white fluffy mustache has crumbs from the late morning snack I must have just interrupted. I feather my finger beneath my nose, hinting at the small mess on his face. The poor man's cheeks redden, and he turns around to retrieve his handkerchief.

"My sincerest apologies, dear. Sometimes I forget to take care of myself at this old age. After my wife, Edna, passed, God bless her soul, I find it hard to look in a mirror as much as I used to. I was quite a looker in my day if you can believe it."

I place my hand on his arm and squeeze gently. "I'm so sorry to hear about your wife—"

"Mr. Jones," he completes my sentence.

"Mr. Jones, I can't imagine how hard it must be without her." I can, in a way. Losing Mom five years ago feels as though nothing could compare. Although the thought of building a life with someone for half a century, then ending up alone must be pure misery.

"Oh, you know, she's just waiting on me to come home when I'm ready. My Edna was always patient with me, even in the afterlife. God knows I'll probably live until I'm a hundred and three."

To come home.

The thought brings a wave of chills across my cheeks. I never thought of life that way. Are we all just waiting in line to get back *home*, where we belong? If that's what life is all about, it's not a surprise Mom went *home* first, waiting on the rest of us. That's the type of person she was—the one to test the waters before we all jumped in behind her. "That's a friendly way to think, Mr. Jones. I shall remember your words. They mean something to me, as well."

"Have you lost someone, dear?"

I release my hand from his arm and readjust my pocketbook over my shoulder. "Yes, unfortunately, I lost my mother, but I'm carrying on for her, you see. I'm living the life she was building, and I'm doing it to make her proud, as it fulfills me to do so."

"You are wise beyond your years, young lady. Keep up the wonderful spirit. And if you need help with anything, let me know." Mr. Jones gives me a wink and a swoosh of his mustache before turning back for the front counter.

When I look at the furniture, I try to imagine myself in a small house with Everett, cooking together, sitting on a loveseat in front of the radio at night. It's funny how simply these imaginary moments blossom in my mind, but I know it could take a trek around the universe to find ourselves in this perfect place. At least there are no expiration dates on time. I'll continue to imagine us at the age we are now, and it will be the only way I will ever see us —young and carefree.

After a lazy stroll around the shop, I stop by the checkout counter. "Thank you for your time, Mr. Jones. I hope you have a lovely day," I offer before lowering my sunglasses down to my nose.

"You, as well, young lady. Thank you for the pleasant chat."

It seems I've lallygagged around long enough this morning, leaving me with just enough time to make it back to Audrey's house for tea. I hoist myself up on the banana seat of my bicycle and stroll by the endlessly long lines of men waiting to enlist, wishing I could put the thoughts in the back of my mind for just a short while, but no matter where I look, there is a reminder of war at every corner and on every street. There is no way to fool myself into thinking everything is normal again.

I pull into Audrey's driveway and settle my bicycle next to hers alongside the garage. I smooth out the wrinkles in my dress and pull my compact out from my purse to check my makeup and hair. Lately, when I see my reflection, I feel like I'm staring at a stranger lost in the middle of two worlds. I don't know how long I'll feel this way, but the unsettling stress is causing puffy shadows beneath my lashes that I can't seem to conceal with makeup. We are all tired and worn out, but it would be nice to see a light at the end of this dark tunnel. I know there won't be such a thing for a long time, though.

I tap my knuckles against the storm door of Audrey's house. Within seconds, she opens the door and welcomes me inside. Our hug feels flimsy today, as if it's something we're supposed to do rather than want to do. "I just put the water on the burner. It should just be a few minutes," she says.

"It's okay. I didn't come for the tea. I'm here to see you, silly."

"Of course," she says. "Can I take your gloves and sweater?"

I slowly peel my gloves off, one finger at a time, then remove my sweater, all while trying to understand the chill I'm getting from Audrey's demeanor.

"This doesn't feel right," I tell her after she hangs up my sweater and places my gloves down neatly on their entryway table.

"What do you mean?"

I perch down on her sofa, a pronounced stiffness in my back is surely proof of my discomfort with our encounter but I'm not sure she's feeling much better, certainly not enough to respond truthfully.

"Well, I'm already aware of your feelings toward my life decisions as of late, but we have always supported each other, and this tension feels more like anger than fear or disappointment. Aside from enlisting in the Army Nurse Corps, did I upset you?" Audrey has often been the type to need space when she's upset. She spins through a cycle of dissecting whatever is bothering her, and until she comes to terms with the situation, she keeps her thoughts to herself. This feels like more, though. It seems to grow worse and worse and has been over the last few months. I was sure she had gotten over my relationship with Everett. She seemed to accept everything once Dad found out, despite his anger of my attempt at keeping Everett a secret.

"I'm not sure how to explain my feelings, Lizzie," she says, taking a seat beside me. We both twist to face each other and when I look into her eyes, I see a flicker of desolation. "Life is changing so fast and I'm having a hard time keeping up, I suppose." Audrey's gaze falls to her folded hands. Her thumbs twiddle back and forth as she pauses between her statements. "First, it was Everett and the stress of keeping a secret that could land you in trouble, and there was little time between your Dad finally learning the truth and then the attack on Pearl. Without a minute to catch our breaths after that, you enlisted in the Army Nurse Corps. Before we know it, you'll be moving away from Hawaii."

I didn't consider Audrey's attitude toward me to be stemming from grief. "You know, no matter where I end up or go, we're always going to be best friends, Audrey. We can call each other or write letters, and of course I'll come home. My family is here, and that includes you."

Audrey drops her hands to her lap with silent exasperation. "It just won't be the same anymore. I realize I have been so focused on becoming a nurse that I have no other friends or prospects in my dating life. And of course, these are all very selfish comments, which is why I have tried to keep quiet about it all, but I'm sad, worried, and scared that you won't be here anymore. We've always been like peas and carrots, you know? I guess I've been trying to distance myself, so it won't be so bad when you leave."

Audrey and I have certainly grown up differently than others, living here on base. People come and go so often that it's rare to have a friend stick around for as long as we have for each other. "We will always be close, Audrey. Nothing can take that away from us. No man, no war, and no job."

A small smile presses into Audrey's cheeks, but the moment of reassurance is concealed by the brassy whistle from the teapot. Audrey hops up from the sofa and tends to the kettle, preparing our two cups. "Could I help?" I offer.

"No, no, I'm all set. Would you like biscotti?"

"Yes, please, that would be lovely." Audrey places the teacups and saucers down on the coffee table in front of the sofa before reclaiming her seat within the indent she left behind. "Have you considered joining the Army Nurse Corps?" I'm sure her reaction toward me joining is the answer to this question, but I'm curious if she has given the idea any thought.

"I have, in fact," she says. "But what are the chances of us being stationed in the same place?" I feel blindsided by her question. It's the last thing I expected to hear. "Oh, I honestly have no clue how or when this all happens. I haven't heard a peep since I filled out my paperwork a few weeks ago. I wasn't aware you were even considering this path. Why haven't you mentioned it to me?" Aside from the fact that we have spent little time together, I would think she might have made a point of bringing it up.

"I'm still struggling with the idea," she says. "Part of me thinks if we were together, I could protect you if times get tough, but after growing up here on the base and seeing all the comings and goings, I'm sure the chances are slim we would end up together."

"Protect me?" I question. "That's not the reason you should consider the Army Nurse Corps, Audrey."

Audrey forces a pause in our conversation as she lifts her teacup and gently blows at the steam before taking a small sip. I do the same for the sake of not staring at her with the million questions running through my mind.

"Lizzie, do you listen to the radio or read the papers? For a girl who has always had her nose in a book, I find it hard to believe you don't see the danger you are potentially facing."

"Wherever I end up, which may be nowhere near Europe, it's because I want to help the wounded and ill. I didn't enlist to start a motion about Jewish Americans," I argue.

"There is an abundance of anti-Semitism growing across the globe, Lizzie. It's the worst in Europe. They have tagged every Jewish person with a yellow star patch and have prohibited them from working or leaving their country. It's beyond anti-Semitism. What if someone were to find out you are Jewish? Would they be able to find out you are Jewish? Do you know the answer to this because I'm guessing you do not?"

I take a moment to process her question and straighten the scarlet tapestry pillow between us. "How would someone find out I'm Jewish?" I reply, sounding as hostile as I feel inside.

"Without intending to be offensive, your last name is easy to decipher its origin, and if someone were to look hard enough, there is religious information on your personal records. It wouldn't be difficult to figure out."

Knowing my last name deciphers my ethnic background has never been something to bother me or make me think it could cause an issue. "Maybe I'll just have to change my last name," I chide.

"If I wasn't already clear on the rules for enlisting in the Nurse Corps, I might think you are crazy enough to run off and marry Everett while you have the chance, but we know that isn't an option. Therefore, changing your last name isn't either. Lizzie, you need to be realistic about what I'm saying. This is a dangerous situation you have put yourself in."

"If I deploy to Europe, yes. If not, I will be fine. Either way, I am an American signing up to help our military in their time of need. This isn't something I want to worry about until I know more about where I will be training. I'm sorry. I appreciate your concern, but there isn't much to worry about at the moment. And I ask that you not enlist for the hope of somehow protecting me from the evils in the world. I love you for thinking like that, but I will be fine. I'm sure of it."

Audrey places her teacup down next to mine on the coffee

table and leans forward to pull me in for an embrace. "I will always worry about you. We're like sisters, and the thought of you being in danger cuts through me at my core."

"This is my destiny, wherever it may be, however long it might last, and whenever it comes to fruition. I need to do this for me."

"I know."

"Think about traveling the world and meeting lots of new people and seeing the sights we could never imagine."

"It doesn't sound like the worst way to spend the next few years, but I'm not one who chases the unknown down a dark road, Lizzie." Audrey laughs to highlight her words as a joke. Though, I know it isn't a joke because it's true and it's the way I prefer to live.

"You do what will make you happy and then when we have found our happiness and peace in the world, we will find each other again and it will be like no time has passed," I say.

Audrey releases her arms from around my neck and pinches her hand around my chin. "I wish you could promise this," she says.

I can only promise today. It's that way for everybody. She knows how I feel about defining a future no one can foresee. I would love to tell her about my guilty little dream of having time to move to Georgia with Everett before I'm assigned to a unit, but I could only imagine what her thoughts would be on that matter, and Everett's overheard orders must remain private for now.

30

JANUARY 1942

THE HOURS of conversation felt like they used to between Audrey and me. I missed the days where we lost track of time while catching up on life, and though we still have our opposing views; I feel like we understand each other better now and I needed that comfort to take with me for whatever comes next — even if it's just supper with Dad, James, and Lewis tonight. Everett has to attend a meeting with his colonel, and he expects it to go past supper time. I assume he's finding out the relocation information that I overheard this morning.

He said he would try to call me later and let me know what happened. At least I can assume it won't be any more shocking than what we're already thinking. Scalloped potatoes, boiled chicken, and green beans — it's been the same several times in the last two weeks. The stores are not replenishing food items and staples in a timely manner or with a good quantity when they do. There's a shortage across the country from what I've heard. A lot of panic will clear the shelves fast. The older generations fearful about another great depression and the younger generations haven't experienced war time yet. Though I'm part of the younger generation, I know all too much of what life was like during the first world war and there was a legitimate reason to stock up on supplies and canned goods. Predicting what will happen the next day is impossible.

"Chicken," Lewis says as he walks through the front door. He removes his cap and hangs it on the coat rack. "I'm sorry, kid. I know you hate chicken."

"It's fine. I'm also making gravy," I tell him.

"You're too good to us, Elizabeth. I don't know what we're going to do without you here."

"Well, at this rate, who knows when I'll be going anywhere. Maybe they passed on my application."

"If that's the case, you'll have time to find out who James's new girlfriend is because I've been trying to figure it out for the last week and he won't even give me a hint. He's not coming home for supper tonight. That's all I know."

"I can only imagine what he has up his sleeve," I reply. James does not have an outstanding track record with women and never brings them home for that exact reason. He finds the lame dames, as Lewis and I call them—the ones who bat their extra-long fake eyelashes and have their bosoms hanging out of whatever outfit they squeeze into. These girls want a sailor, and they are not shy about going after one. The hot tickets end up being a young eighteen-year-old daughter of a sailor or soldier.

"There's a chance she could differ from his usual selection. Heck, maybe that's the reason he's keeping her a secret from us."

"It's not like we embarrass him," I respond, "not all that much, anyway." I can't help but snicker. Maybe we pick on James more than he picks on either of us, but there isn't much else siblings are good for.

We place the jokes on pause when Dad walks through the door. Until we know what kind of mood he's in or what type of day he had, we tread with caution.

"What's that in your hand?" Lewis asks.

I didn't notice the envelope in his hand when he walked in through the door, but it doesn't look like work he'd bring home— not something sealed up the way it is.

"What's in my hand?" Dad repeats, then removes his cover to hang up next to the other on the coat rack. "This is what Elizabeth has been awaiting." Dad walks up to the kitchen table and drops the envelope on top of the hot plate where I plan to put the chicken. The contents create a loud slap which breaks me free from my stare at the enclosed documents. "Go ahead. The envelope contains your orders." Dad's tone sounds like a lesson in the making, and my stomach reels with nerves as I take the couple of steps over to the table. I retrieve the official envelope and slide my finger beneath the seal. My heart is pounding with anticipation, eagerness, and a dose of fear. It hasn't felt quite real until this moment.

"Do you already know what's inside this envelope?" I ask Dad.

"It doesn't matter," he responds.

I pull the papers out and scan down the top sheet. "I will report to Fort Devens in Massachusetts for active duty and training with the 2nd Evacuation Hospital on January 21," I speak aloud as I read the information, trying to digest the words, and meaning. *January 21*. I step into the kitchen and lean toward the new Coca-Cola calendar I gave Dad for Hanukkah a few weeks ago. "The date is just a week and a half away—a week from Wednesday."

Dad takes the papers from my hand and scans them as if needing confirmation. He nods his head as I watch his eyes moving from left to right over and over until I flip to the second page I hadn't gotten to yet. I shouldn't be in a state of shock. At least, I shouldn't be acting as if I'm in a state of shock. I knew this was coming. I volunteered.

I'm most likely leaving before Everett has to go.

The cloud of dreamy images of Everett and I living together for a bit evaporates into a mist.

This is what I wanted.

This is what I want.

But my stomach hurts and my chest feels tight.

"You will fly to Boston on January 19th, and from there, take a charter bus to Fort Devens," Dad adds to what I read, reiterating the time I will have to leave. "Well, at least we can celebrate your birthday before you go."

Lewis steps up behind me and wrenches his bear claws around my shoulders. "The baby of the family is turning twenty-one. How is it possible?" I haven't given my birthday much thought. It doesn't feel very significant with everything going on, but now I suppose whatever celebration I have, it will be a going away party too. "You can finally purchase beer and wine. How about that?"

Dad clears his throat as if Lewis has gone too far with his celebratory ideas. "Let's not start any bad habits a week before you leave for training."

"Dad, it's her twenty-first birthday. We aren't letting the kid leave without a proper celebration," Lewis argues.

"It's not a big deal."

"This training looks like it might be intense, Elizabeth. You should start exercising over the next few days to prepare yourself more."

"I have been jogging almost daily for the last few weeks," I tell him. "I am well aware of what I signed up for, despite what you might think."

"Well, you are bone pale for someone who knows for certain what they volunteered for," Dad continues. The paperwork falls from his hand, fanning out against the table before he retreats to his bedroom without another word.

"He will get over it, Elizabeth, because he would be a hypocrite if he didn't." Dad's biggest pet peeve is being a hypocrite. Lewis has a good point.

"I'm a woman and his daughter. In his mind, I don't think he sees me the same as one of you."

"Give it time. The world is changing at full speed right now. He will have to come to terms with reality sooner rather than later. For the record, though, I'm proud of you. I'm going to miss you like crazy, but I always had this little suspicion in the back of my head, you would be the first in our family to make a giant leap into the turn of the century."

"Mom was a nurse too," I remind him.

"Sure, for the Red Cross, which is more than noble, but you've taken things a step further. You are the first woman in our family to enlist in the military, Elizabeth. This is a big deal."

I wonder if what I'm feeling is natural. Adrenaline carried me through the door to the Red Cross. Pride escorted me home with the explanation I was honored to stand up for. Now, panic is ensuing from thoughts about a tomorrow, the day after that, and so on. I can no longer live one day at a time. Now I must face what lies ahead: all the warnings I have been digesting for the last few weeks.

31

JANUARY 1942

WHEN I THINK BACK to the anticipation leading up to this day, like everyone else my age, I was looking forward to my twenty-first birthday. I imagined a wild party on the beach with a bonfire while welcoming the newfound sense of freedom. At eighteen a person becomes a legal adult under state laws, which allows men and women to vote and men to enlist in the military. At twenty-one, I'm now allowed to drink alcohol and join the Army Nurse Corps, but the only thing that feels different from all the days drawing closer to the special milestone in my life, are my nerves.

I'm sure once Everett arrives, I'll be able to put my racing thoughts to the side for a bit and enjoy what I can of the day. I promised Dad we could have a family dinner later tonight, and he even offered to cook something up, which frightens me a little. It's the thought that counts, though.

With my bright floral sundress and matching navy-blue bolero, I feel ready to enjoy the warm sun and mild breeze. After receiving my orders last week, I fleetingly came to realize how much sun I should soak up before leaving for the Northeast. When I arrive in Massachusetts, I believe the temperatures will be below freezing. I'm not sure what that will feel like having grown up in a tropical paradise, but I imagine it will take some adjusting. I must have spent a minute too long inspecting the shade of strawberry-red lipstick I colored over my lips because the doorbell makes me jump, causing a slight smudge of the top right corner on my lip. *Just wonderful.* I snag my handkerchief from the top of my vanity and dab away the stain. The doorbell rings again, proving impatience or perhaps eagerness. Mom always told me it was important to make a man wait sometimes, but it's something I have a hard time with.

I grab my white low heel peep-toe pumps and run for the door, opening it with a flurry of anticipation, finding a magnificent bouquet held out in front of Everett's face. My favorite fragrant sunshine-yellow plumerias surrounded by sweet scented pink ginger and towering lobster orange heliconia. I wish my first thought isn't whether I can bring these along with me on the plane next week. The second thought is to take them from Everett's hand so I can kiss the beautiful man who thinks so dearly of me today. "My, oh my, I believe you might just be the sweetest man alive," I tell him.

With a soft prideful grin, he drops his gaze as if embarrassed by my comment but resets his eyes on mine immediately. "Happy Birthday, doll-face."

"Thank you," I coo. "These are beautiful." I take another whiff before making my way into the kitchen to retrieve a vase from beneath the sink. "I don't think I've ever received something so extravagant for a birthday. You sure know how to spoil a girl, Everett."

"I wouldn't call this spoiling you. You deserve the world, baby?"

His words settle in my head as I twist the faucet knob to fill the vase. I remove the paper wrapping and lower the stems into the freshwater. "Perfect," I say, spinning around to face Everett. He appears troubled while staring out the bay window. "You know, even if you just showed up with a smile today, it would have been more than enough for me. You know me better than to wish for extravagance."

"There is a difference between what you may wish for and what I believe you deserve. And you, Miss Elizabeth, deserve the whole universe."

"Part of me feels as though you've already given that to me and then some," I reply.

"This is only the beginning. I can promise you that. This—us —it's only going to get better from here on out, distance or not, nothing will keep me from showing you how much love I feel for you every day."

Everett holds his hand out for me to take. It's such a sweet, simple gesture, but when he takes my hand and curls me into his arms, I feel like he is the universe and I'm the core of it all. How could I want anything more? He places a kiss on my cheek and releases his arms to reopen the front door. "Are you ready for a special outing?"

I tap my finger against my lips. "Hmm, I'm not sure. I'm the one who typically plans the surprises, and now I don't know if I enjoy being the one who doesn't know what's happening."

"Well, gosh, that's just too bad for you. Come on, let's get out of here, doll." I slip my shoes on as we walk out the door, and I lock up as Everett holds the storm door open for me. "By the way, you look gorgeous today." I swat at the sleeve of his forest green uniform jacket.

"You are so smooth, you know that?"

"With only a week left before you leave, I must get in all the compliments I can now so you have something to think about when you take off."

"What about you? How will I be able to do the same in a couple weeks when you're getting ready to move down to Georgia?"

"You've given me enough to dream about for a lifetime, sweetheart."

I know he didn't mean to bring the mood down, regarding us both leaving Oahu, but I feel like I just got hit in the chest by a splash of frozen water. I've always been good at putting reality to the side, but when it's brought up to me, it's a raw reminder of what I'm facing —what I volunteered for. I can't comment with a complaint or even a sigh. This was my decision and I have no choice but to stand by it now, regardless of my slight thoughts of regret. I'm sure everyone must feel the same way before embarking on a journey like this one.

We make our way over to Everett's polished car and he opens the passenger side door like always, waiting for me to slide in as if I'm a royal princess. Princesses don't enlist in the Army though. It is why I have done what I have. I am not a princess, nor do I want to portray one.

Once the engine roars to life, Everett turns the volume knob to the right. There's static for a moment as he pulls away from my house, but as we near the end of the street, one of my favorite songs plays through the speakers. It's Frank Sinatra singing, *"I'll Never Smile Again."* The reminder is perfect for the moment.

"Everett," I say above the music.

He peers over at me for a brief second. "Why the pout, baby?"

"What if the lyrics to this song are true? What if I can never smile, laugh, or feel a thrill again until I'm back with you? You have brought me so much joy over the last eight months. I didn't want to admit this out loud to you or anyone, but I'm nervous and a bit terrified to leave."

Everett reaches across the leather bench of the seat and places his hand on top of mine. "You are following your life's purpose and our love can survive until you prove to yourself and everyone else, how worthy you are. I promise you will find reasons to smile and laugh each day because you find the good in every part of life."

"You're the good in my life," I follow.

"I am only one or part of the 'good' you're speaking about. I know this change is scary—change is always frightening, but it's exhilarating too. You are setting off on an adventure that will bring you a feeling of achievement. You can't go through life ignoring your needs because that is where regret begins. From there, it will sink its claws in, leaving you to question all your decisions."

He is repeating the sentiments I have expressed to him, but in different words. He's right, and I was too. "Say, where do you think you're going?" I ask, noticing we're driving in the opposite direction of downtown.

"You'll see," he says, throwing me a quick wink.

I drum my fingertips against the pleats on my skirt as

excitement masks my apprehension. "Why, you're taking me to the beach, aren't you?" I gush. "Of course, you are. Where else would I want to spend my birthday? This is simply perfect, Everett. Thank you."

"Shh," he says. "I haven't heard you say so much with so much enthusiasm since the week we first met. You really are a bundle of nerves, huh?"

I clear my throat and clasp my hands over my lap. "I will be fine."

"You certainly will be. And in three weeks from now, when I'm getting ready to head down to Fort Benning in Georgia, I'll be feeling the same way. You should have seen me the week before I left Los Angeles to fly here. I was a head case and had already been through the rigorous training. I think I came to realize it wasn't a bad type of stress—it was a new type of hunger for unfamiliar territory."

I smile at his explanation as it clarifies what I'm feeling—less fear and more impatience for something new. The car jerks around as we roll over the rubble covered parking lot amidst a mess of large lava rocks and tangled vines of greenery—a bit of our natural habitat that didn't burn to ashes.

Everett takes my hand as we descend the uneven pathway to the beach. "I would have chosen better shoes to wear, had I known," I tell him, holding on with my tightest grip.

"Knowing you, your shoes will be off those cute feet of yours in a matter of seconds anyway." I suppose I can't help the free-spirited person I grew up to be on this island, despite my strict upbringing. If I could live barefoot on the sand and sleep against the ocean's edge, I would. *Maybe someday.*

"Surprise!" Dozens of voices jolt me into losing my footing in the sand, but Everett must have known it was coming and had a good hold on me as I would have likely fallen to my face.

I clutch my free hand against my chest, finding all the familiar faces I love. "Happy Birthday, Elizabeth!"

My mouth falls open and I can't figure out how to wipe the shocked look from my face. I've never had a surprise party. "You're all here," I say.

"Where else would we be today?" Audrey asks, running

toward me with a red hibiscus lei dangling from her wrists. "Hau'oli Lā Hānau—Happy Birthday, my best friend." She places a string necklace threaded through flowers around my neck.

"Did you have something to do with this?" I ask.

She pinches her fingers against my cheek. "Well, let's see here. A beach fire, some music pumping out of our car speakers, and a little luau with your favorite foods."

"For me? You did this all for me?"

"We all did," Audrey says. "We all love you."

Dad, James, and Lewis make their way over to me and squeeze me into a family bear hug that leaves me coughing for air. "I don't know how my little girl is this old, but you better make it stop right now, you hear me?" Dad is in a hula shirt for the second time in years, and he looks relaxed, not as uptight as he's been.

I spot Audrey's parents, Mr. and Mrs. Evens, and a couple of Everett's friends who I have become fond of over the past few months. They're chatting away with a couple of my girlfriends from nursing school. Then I notice a face I don't recognize. She appears to be native to the island, unlike the rest of us. She's a beautiful woman with waist length shimmering midnight black hair, a tan I would do anything for, and a small narrow frame. I have no clue who she is.

"Who is that woman?" I ask, speaking over Dad and Everett.

They both look over in the direction I'm staring and furrow their brows. "I do not know. Did she just get here?" Dad asks.

"Oh, that's uh—that there is, Lokelani."

"That's swell, James, but who is Lokelani?" Lewis presses.

"Easy, easy, don't flip your wig, okay?" James says, taking a step in toward us.

"Aw, look how slack happy he is. That's the girl," I say, maybe a touch louder than intended.

"Lay off. Look. I don't want to scare her away, okay. She's a good girl and already overwhelmed. So, can you just try to be nice and not ask her a million questions tonight, maybe?"

I throw my hands on top of James's shoulders. "My big brother, why would I do something silly like ask the poor girl a million questions tonight? It's not like I'm leaving and might come home to a new sister-in-law or something. Oh wait, I am leaving, and you have been hiding a woman from us, which can only mean one thing."

Lewis falls into a fit of laughter. "You are head over heels in love with this broad, aren't you?"

"This is the first we're hearing about this girl, James? What's in the world is the meaning of this?" Dad asks.

It's nice not to be the one everyone is darting their eyes at for a change, and it might be the perfect opportunity to go meet this poor girl. I wonder if anyone has warned her about James needing a human alarm buzzer to wake up in the morning, or that he can't avoid burning toast if his life were to depend on it. Heck, I'm not sure he even knows how to plug a vacuum cleaner in, but maybe she's okay with that. I'll ease her in gently.

"Elizabeth, take it easy on her please," Dad says. "You are leaving, and it would be nice for James to find someone else to wake him up in the mornings."

"This is great. Thanks," James says, grumbling on his way back over to Lokelani.

"I'll go over first. I'm more subtle than you two," Lewis says to Dad and me.

"This conversation has just made me realize how hard I should think before I consider joining this family someday," Everett says with a sigh.

"It's too late, son. You're already one of us. Once you break down the barrier, there's no going back and I hate to say it, but I like you too much, kid. You aren't going anywhere. You understand?"

"Yes, Sir," Everett responds, saluting Dad out of habit after speaking the word "sir."

Dad slaps Everett's arm down. "I warned you about that, son. You do not need to salute me when we're off duty."

"Yes, Sir."

I elbow him in the gut. "Stop it," I mumble.

"I'm going to change out of my uniform at the bathroom up the hill. I'll be back in a few minutes, doll. Please don't get yourself in any trouble while I'm gone."

"And that is why I like this man," Dad says.

Go figure I find a man Dad wants to call his son and I sign my life away for God knows how long.

THE AIRPORT: a place of hellos and goodbyes.

I thought the days would go by in a blink this past week, but they crawled by, minute to minute, and hour to hour—every second consumed with "what ifs." There were moments when I thought someone might reach out and tell me they made a mistake in assigning me orders, or that I wasn't skilled enough to take part in something so prestigious, but none of that happened. I'm here at the airport, preparing to say goodbye to my family, Audrey, and Everett, and I don't know when I'll see them again, or if I will see them again? It's part of one of my "what ifs."

Dad is not good with goodbyes. He never has been. It's always quick, gutting, and we move on, but that's only been for when he's leaving on a deployment. He isn't any stronger when Lewis or James ever leaves either. His love for us runs deep, and seemingly painful sometimes.

"Listen to me, kiddo, don't let anyone give you crap. Keep your head up, your mind straight, and do what you're good at doing," James tells me.

"Talking?" I joke.

"Maybe you could try to do a little less of that in this case," he continues.

It isn't often when James acts sensitive to anything, except recently, he seems to have found himself a weakness named

Lokelani. It's like someone turned on a lightbulb and he can suddenly understand the inner workings of a woman's brain. One might think after living with his sister for twenty-one years he'd have it figured out, but it took this woman to make him see straight. She is one of the sweetest, gentlest people I have ever met, and I don't know what she sees in my brother, but I hope she feels the same way about him. "And you, James, don't mess up with Lokelani. I like her and I'm glad we got the chance to meet. She's incredible."

James's cheeks brighten into a scarlet hue, and it might be the first time in history I have embarrassed my brother. I will call it a win.

"I'll try," he says. "Take care of yourself, Lizzie. I'll miss you. Don't forget to write. You know the rules."

"I know the rules. Once a week or someone is coming after me," I say repeating the words Dad has always said to James and Lewis before they take off for a mission.

James gives me a quick wink and squeezes the air out of my lungs with his bear claws.

Lewis is next and I can already see a red stain forming within the whites of his eyes. He won't cry, but he will come close to sucking back a tear if need be. "I don't know how this is even happening right now," he says. "I'm going to miss you so much."

Lewis repeats James's motion of embracing me to where I gasp for air. He's shorter on words than James when he's hurting or upset. I assume Dad's speech will be even shorter.

Before I have the chance to look in his direction, his arms are already around me and he buries his face into my shoulder. "Please come home in one piece, Elizabeth. Please. I have faith in you, in everything you put your mind too. Just don't let your heart impede your head and you'll be fine. You understand?"

"I do," I mutter, feeling the heaviness in my chest bear down against my aching heart.

"Those letters, Elizabeth. Don't you dare forget, and if you can call me, you call me, at work or at home—whenever possible."

If I open my mouth to talk, a sob might escape, so I swallow the lump in my throat and nod my head. Dad turns his cheek and kisses my temple. "God, I love you so much, sweetheart. I'm proud of you. Never forget."

As if a bolt of lightning strikes us both, Dad walks away and is out of sight, escaping from a heart-wrenching scene. Lewis gives me a quick wave and follows in the direction Dad must have gone.

"Love you, kid," James says, turning to follow Lewis.

I didn't think this could get much worse, but Audrey is in a mess of tears and I can't make out a word of what she's saying as she throws her arms around my neck. "Tell me if you find someone for me out in Massachusetts. Maybe it'll entice me to come out there to keep an eye on you," she mumbles through her choking cries.

I laugh at her pathetic sounding statement. "I promise to keep an eye out for eligible bachelors that are suitable for you."

Everett clears his throat to remind me of his proximity and likely the words about keeping my eye open for other men. He's smiling, but it's an act I can see right through.

"Love you, Lizzie," Audrey moans. Everett hands her a handkerchief, and she scuffles off toward the exit.

I'm not sure my heart can take much more right now, but it's buckling, bringing me to a new level of weakness. "Come on, I'll walk you to the gate."

I want Everett to come with me. I've changed my mind. I want to settle down, get married, and have a family. I'll cook, clean, and do what I'm supposed to do if it means staying with him.

My thoughts come and go as we pass another Army Nurse Corps recruiting sign with the words, "We Need You" written in sharp red letters. The message is loud and clear. I'm not housewife material—I've been preparing for more, more than I think I can handle.

"I don't think I have ever heard you this quiet, Lizzie. In fact, you're so quiet, I think I hear the words screaming through your head." I glance over at the green eyes I adore, giving him my best doe-eyed stare back. "Don't do that. You'll crush me too."

"Don't do what?" I ask, playing along.

"Don't look at me like I'm breaking your heart." At this moment, I'm the heartbreaker.

"You could never do such a thing. I—I just have to admit, I didn't think this would be as hard as it is."

"Well, changing the world for the better, there's nothing easy about it, but you're leading the way for other strong women, Elizabeth, and with all the other thoughts of discontentment and sadness put to the side, look at how far you've come to get to this moment. Your mother would stand here with her shoulders straight and pride glistening through her eyes that match yours. You are succeeding at something women for generations will come to know you for. You will be their guiding light and you'll show them they can reach for the stars and grab them all."

His words are the reason I'm here. His words have been constant thoughts since Mom passed away. If I don't leave my footprint behind for Mom and me, I will have wasted a perfectly good life.

Everett is quiet for the few minutes it takes to move across the terminal. As the gate unfurls into sight, my stomach drops lower and lower. "Was it worth it?" I ask. I'm not sure if he understands what I'm asking, but I'm having trouble coming up with the right words to explain myself.

Everett takes me by the wrist and stops me from walking forward. "Did you just ask me if 'it' was worth it?" I nod in agreement. "If the 'it' you are referring to is 'you,' Elizabeth, then I refuse to answer such a question." Maybe he doesn't intend to answer me, but it doesn't appear he plans to release his grip either. "You know what, no, if you need an answer, I'll give you one." He swallows hard and shakes his head with frustration crinkling into fine lines on his forehead. "From the second you almost took an entire aisle of shelving units down at the commissary and I turned the corner to see this beautiful mess of a girl trying to fix her mistake, I knew there was something special about you. It's why I came up to you while you were waiting at the checkout counter. You drew me in, and I may never know why, but I'm sure glad I followed my gut. Heck, I'm even glad I got this scar on my face a week later because it meant you got to stick a needle and thread into my Hollywood profile." Only Everett could bring humor to a moment like this. "You have been worth every single second I have spent on this island, every horrific minute endured over the last couple months, every sleepless night when I couldn't be with you, and every moment you stole my breath when I was with you. If you were to walk away from me right here, right now with a forever goodbye, I'd still say it was worth it."

I can't cry. If I pop that cork, it will be a mess of an explosion in the middle of the airport. "Everett," I say, trying to interrupt him from saying anything more that will make me break.

"But then I'll go outside with the rest of your family and cry like a child who dropped his ice cream cone on a hot day."

I snicker, pushing the tears back for another quick second. "Will we both come back home?" Neither of us can answer this question, but I need him to lie right now.

"Yes, Lizzie, we're both coming home from this. And until then, when you need me, you can look up to the sky and find a cloud that represents the sign or reassurance you're looking for because that'll be the same cloud I will be flying through at that same moment. If you look hard enough, you'll see me waving." He's awfully good at this goodbye and I am failing on holding up my end.

"Well, please just watch where you're going and no loop-de-loops like you tell me about. Oh, and if you end up lost somehow, don't go flying to the moon without me or anything. That's not part of your job," I remind him—the man with eyes set out to see this world from space while settling for a spot within the clouds.

"I won't go to the moon with you, baby."

Finally, we're both smiling. We're both masking the pain with words neither can promise, but it's what we need. "That's fair, but if I got rules, so do you. Don't pick fights with someone you can't take and keep some of your thoughts to yourself. Just some, okay, doll?"

I hold out my other hand to shake on the deal, and he takes my hand and pulls me in against his chest. His palms cup my cheeks, and he leans down ever so slowly, as snaillike as this last week has gone, and gently touches his lips to mine. I inhale the memory and the scent of his love, knowing something this strong will never fade away. "I love you," he whispers against my lips.

"Always," I murmur.

"And forever ... Don't forget that part," he says.

"Of course, I won't forget."

Everett reaches into his pocket and pulls out a photograph I took early last summer. "I have this for you—put this in your journal and don't read the words on the back unless you are sure the worst has come for us and you are desperate for a reminder of why you're doing what you're doing." The photograph is my favorite of him. We were at the beach. The wind was blowing like crazy and the sun was illuminating his eyes. It was a perfect moment to capture.

"I love this picture," I say, forcing my eyes to part with the reminder of a wonderful moment. "I have one for you too with a little note in case you need a reminder of how much I love you in between letters and phone calls."

I retrieve the small envelope from the front of my pocketbook and hand it to him, showing off the kiss mark I left on the flap.

He holds it up to his nose and closes his eyes. "Your perfume —you—you are just perfect."

33

JANUARY 1942

THE PAPERS with my orders contained a bus number to locate once I arrived in Boston. I'm unsure if the bus is only for Fort Devens personnel or if I will arrive somewhere near Fort Devens. There isn't any further information other than the mode of transportation. Maybe I'll be able to catch a few minutes of sleep on this bus because I feel as though I have been traveling for two days straight and could not nap on the plane. The chatter from the surrounding seats never ceased, even from the dark hours to the moment the morning sun peeked over the horizon.

I spent most of my hours staring out the window, feeling grateful I wasn't sitting between the other two men in my row of seats. The clouds held my unwavering focus as I realized how much closer I felt to mom. I know heaven isn't in the clouds, but I found a small sense of comfort while looking out at the white fog, wondering if she could see me from the other side. I imagined skipping along the balls of white cotton and watching the world spin below.

Several times, I reached into my purse to retrieve my journal, wanting to write, but each time, I realized I was at a loss for words. I have only seen the clouds and a swarm of people occupying seats around me and no one communicating with me since I left home. I think it was the newfound sense of loneliness that left me with nothing but empty thoughts, paper, and a pen.

While waiting for the bus to depart from the airport, I glance around, spotting more empty seats than filled ones. No one appears to be looking for a conversation. Everyone is quiet and either reading a paper, book, or staring out the window. In Oahu, it's hard to find someone who isn't eager to start a conversation with anyone on the street. It could be as mundane as the temperature of the ocean, but there is no shortage of people to keep one from feeling alone.

I pull my wool coat tighter over my chest, feeling a draft move down the aisle. I noticed the snow-covered landscape while landing. From above, it looked more like a white blanket covering the state of Massachusetts. It's the first time I've seen snow, and it's as beautiful as I imagined. However, it is much colder than I imagined too.

The hum of the bus motor and the silence between the seats allows me the comfort to close my eyes for a bit. According to my map, we are forty miles away from Fort Devens. I can assume the bus might take a while to arrive. What's another couple of hours of travel after coming this far?

The accordion door squeals and moans as the driver pulls the crank. Finally, we'll be on our way. A bit of commotion stirs among the first few rows of seats, and before I have the chance to open my eyes, the seat beside me becomes occupied by a person trying to catch their ragged breaths.

"I did not think I was going to make it. Lord almighty."

I'm unsure if this woman is speaking to herself or me, but I offer the common courtesy of peering over.

"Is everything all right?" I ask.

"My plane arrived late, and I don't know if there's another bus leaving Boston for Ayer today."

"I had the same concern," I explain.

"Evidently Ayer is such a small little town that there aren't many people looking to catch a ride there. I don't think there's much to do in the area. At least that's what I've heard. Are you visiting someone or going home? Gosh, where are my manners. I'm Betsy Belson. I know. What were my parents thinking? Well, they weren't, and twenty-two years later I am still dealing with the repercussion of my given name. I just ask people to call me

BB. It's much easier and less mortifying. How about you? What's your name?"

It's hard to believe I have met someone who speaks more words in a minute than I do. It must be a miracle. However, now I know what everyone else must feel like when listening to me. Maybe I don't sound as wound up, though. I slip my glove off my right hand to offer a handshake. "I'm Elizabeth Salzberg, Lizzie, and I'm from Hawaii reporting to Fort Devens for nursing duties."

"Hawaii, huh? Well, that sure explains the beautiful tan against a blonde head of hair," Betsy says, shaking my hand. "You must have been traveling for days at this point. I've heard the flight from the East coast to Hawaii is brutally long." Betsy takes a breath but only for what seems like half of a second. "I'm also reporting to nursing duties at Fort Devens. But I haven't come from as far away as you have. I'm from Cleveland in Ohio, so the travel hasn't been too bad." I'm becoming dizzy listening to her speak so fast as I try to keep up with every word. Even her dark curls bounce against the tops of her shoulders along with each word. She pulls out a tube of lipstick from her purse and applies the red pigment without a compact or a breath in her conversation.

"It's nice to meet someone else reporting to Fort Devens," I offer. It is. I was worried everyone might already know one another, and it would feel like the first day at a new school. I was lucky to avoid moving around like most military children do, but there were changes here and there and times I had to be the new girl. It was never my favorite feeling.

"No kidding, I hate being the new girl in town, you know?" Betsy has a sharp edge to her attitude and demeanor, but I suppose it could be a welcoming change from the uptight lifestyle I'm coming from. She also seems better prepared than I am. Her tweed wool coat is much thicker than mine and her stockings look as though they keep the chill off her skin. She's wearing loafers and Bobby socks, and I'm in heels. She's better prepared for the frigid northeast winter than I am.

"Wait a minute. You said you are from Hawaii. Were you there when the attack on Pearl Harbor happened?"

No one has asked me a question about that day at Pearl. In Oahu, we were all there and had unique experiences but there was never a need to hear other points of view. It's too painful to recall the details and nothing anyone wanted to hear when it felt like we were still living the aftermath day after day. "I was there for the attack. It was dreadful."

"Oh my gosh, I can't even imagine. It's just unimaginable. I probably shouldn't have mentioned the reminder."

I wave her words off with a flick of my wrist. "Oh, please, don't be silly. I'm perfectly fine."

Betsy places her hand over her chest, still seemingly affected by my statement, but she continues with the questions anyway. "Do you still have family in Hawaii?"

"My father and brothers are in the Navy and have been stationed in Oahu most of my life."

"Ah, you're a military brat. You must already know what you're in for then, huh?" Maybe the look in my eyes in response to her question has stopped her from furthering her interrogation of me, or maybe she isn't sure what to ask, but it's clear the subject is changing, appreciatively so.

I slip my glove back on my hand and clasp my fingers together, resting them on my lap. "I have an idea, yes. What about you? Are any of your family members enlisted?"

"Heck no, my mother is an alcoholic and my father is a used car salesman. We've lived in a trailer for the last five years and this was an opportunity for me to get out of Cleveland. I figure nothing can be much worse than being almost twenty-two and living in a dump with my parents." Betsy pulls a cigarette case and a matchbook out of her coat pocket. The metal clicks as it opens, and she holds the full display out to me.

"No, thank you."

She retrieves a cigarette and lights a match. With the red cherry illuminating the curve of her hand she waves the match out and relaxes back into her seat. "I heard the men at Fort Devens are quite fond of the nurses on base. At least that's something to think about, right?"

"Oh, no, not for me—I have a boyfriend back home, Everett. In fact, he's also enlisted in the Army. He's a pilot." My heart thuds at the mention of his name. I didn't expect to feel pain from being away so soon. I've barely had a chance to miss him, but I do. No one has ever snuck into my life so deeply before. This is what I get for letting my guard down with Everett and inviting him into my heart, but I'd rather endure this relentless ache in my chest than to have never known what true love feels like.

"Oh, honey, you can't be serious about a boyfriend across the country. How is that going to work out? Are you two planning on being pen pals or something?"

"We'll do what it takes, I suppose."

"If you want my advice, which you probably don't since I see the lovesick look in your eyes after just a couple days, but I would end it now before it gets too tough. Hey, if you two are meant to be, you'll find each other again someday, right? Plus, with the selection of so many lonely soldiers on base looking for some companionship of the female persuasion, what else are we going to do in our spare time?" Betsy winks and nudges me in the shoulder while blowing out a mouthful of smoke.

I'm not sure how she sees our future turning out, but I doubt we will have much free time, if any at all. However, I know better than to offer my two cents on a subject like this. "I guess we'll just have to wait and see," I respond.

"Do you have a photograph of him? You can't leave a girl hanging. Any man worth waiting for must have something no other guy has."

I debate pulling the photograph out of my breast pocket. Most women know of Everett Anderson. The likelihood of being his girlfriend is so slim she would likely call my story a bluff.

"Oh, it's packed away in my suitcase." If I were to see Everett's face right at this moment, I might break down into a blubbering mess. He wrote me a note on the back side of the photograph and told me not to read the words until I hit rock bottom and need to hear them. I would expect a thunder of laughter from Everett if he knew I couldn't make it off the bus before needing to read his words. Although, for all I know, he may have already read what I wrote to him on the back of my photograph.

The only benefit of listening to Betsy ramble for over an hour is the fact that it made the ride feel shorter than it would have. We pull up to a bus station where I spot two soldiers in uniform waiting stiff as boards with their hands clasped behind their backs. "I wonder how many of us are on this bus?" Betsy mutters as she spots the men too.

As I descend the steps of the bus, I detest that one soldier looks staggeringly like Everett. It must be my imagination, but the sight of him only makes my chest hurt more.

A group of women, all who appear a little lost, seem to appear one by one within a few feet of Betsy and me. All of us have our attention set on the soldiers. Once the bus departs from the station, the soldier who does not look like Everett shouts: "2nd Evacuation, report here for duty." His voice is loud, hoarse, and daunting. Everett's carbon copy places the tips of his fingers against his lips and whistles toward a bus parked several yards away down the curb.

"Welcome to the Army Nurse Corps where you are now reporting for duty on behalf of the United States Army. You must obey every rule and order from this point forward. Any behavior disregarding the policies will be a cause for disciplinary action. Line your suitcases up along the edge of the curb and board the bus that will take you to Fort Devens."

I should be familiar to this tone; the volume of the spoken words, and the meaning—so uncompromising and harsh. I've lived with this familiarity my entire life, but hearing the words directed at me sends an unwavering jolt of unease through my nerves. Being a girl who has never liked to follow rules and got away with doing things I shouldn't have been doing, this transition might be more challenging than I originally thought.

34

JANUARY 1942

THE SECOND BUS trip was not nearly as exhilarating as the one from the airport. We waited for about an hour until the bus departed for Fort Devens. No one spoke a peep through the fifteen-minute ride. I can only imagine that everyone has the same thoughts and questions running through their mind that I do. Though I've grown up in this lifestyle, around military personnel, I'm unsure how different this branch of the Army will be. Women have been enlisting as nurses in the Army since the first World War, but there are so few Army Corps nurses across the country that everything involved seems like classified information. I suspect the number of enlisted nurses is on the rise after the attack on Pearl. It's a new day now, and everything is different, but I'll bet everyone is wondering what comes next.

As I stand in the center of the chaos, I feel dumbstruck. I glance in every direction watching personnel perform tasks and duties, but while there is a consistent movement along the perimeter of the base, there are also several sets of straight-faced stares reciting rules and regulations, directions, assignments, expectations, and timelines. It's will be impossible to remember every word of what I'm listening to, but I'm sure I'm not the only one feeling overwhelmed.

Through the corner of my eyes, I glance at some other faces to my left and right. There are plenty of pale complexions, wide eyes, and fidgeting hands. All these women have been through the rigorous training of becoming a registered nurse over the last few years, but this is different. It will be far more intense and will require not only strong mental cognition but will be physically demanding as well.

"Basic training will begin tomorrow morning at zero five hundred hours here in the quad where you will receive assignments for particular units that will ultimately prepare you for whatever challenges lie ahead."

Captain Landry, our direct report, clasps her gloved hands together in front of her navy-blue wool jacket and matching skirt. On a freshly fallen patch of snow, I assume she must be frigid in her stockings and shiny black laced Oxford shoes standing on the frozen platform, although she is standing stiff as a board. I'm shivering and my muscles are so tight I'm afraid I won't be able to move once we're dismissed. I've never felt cold like this before. My blood needs to thicken up a bit.

"If any of you have questions for me, now is a good time to ask."

The air is distinct here too; it seems thicker and dense with scents I'm not used to. The combination of gunpowder, nicotine, cigar smoke, and coffee beans don't mix well, but I suppose I will become accustomed to it all quickly, especially after having to adapt to the smell of burning metal, wood, and oil-ridden ocean water that had become the normal fragrance in Oahu after the attack.

It shouldn't come as a surprise when Betsy raises her hand with a question. None of the other women seem to have the nerve to open their mouths at the moment. Nor do I. I'm confident we'll find out everything we need to in due time. Captain Landry peers down at her clipboard, then sets her focus on Betsy. "Yes, Second Lieutenant Belson."

"Ah, yeah, I'm just wondering if we'll be able to take a tour of the base at any point. Are any of the nice soldiers walking around available to show us around to help us get acquainted?"

There are muffled sounds of snickers growing from behind gloves or coat sleeves. Captain Landry does not look amused by Betsy's question.

"When there is a need for you to become familiar with each part of this base, you will become acquainted as needed," Captain Landry responds. There is an edge of irritation lacing her words, but by the smirk on Betsy's face, I don't think she's picking up on the obvious cues. Being respectful to rank is a given no matter what service or division a person is in. I would think anyone would know something so simple, but evidently not.

Once Captain Landry completes her introductions, she sends us to a bulletin board adhered to one of the nearby buildings. It's where we will find our room assignments. The women rush to view the list, most of us eager to find some warmth inside the barracks. I wait my turn, trying to be patient as each woman slides her gloved finger down the column of names.

There are only a few different assigned spaces, and the map beside the list shows the direction of mine. It isn't a far walk and I arrive in a large galley room covered in wooden plank floors and raw beams between each mattress covered cot. A handful of black pane windows let in very little light, but the area is brightened from the white ceilings and walls. Each bed has a green wool blanket, a rolled pillow, a pair of wall cabinets with a rod beneath for hanging clothes, and a black studded trunk in front of each metal bed frame. It appears there will be sixteen of us living in these quarters.

A few women are inspecting each corner, the bare cabinets and the trunks waiting for our few personal items we could bring. One woman is checking the firmness of a mattress and curls her lip into a grimace. "It's like a prison, isn't it?" she asks.

This room is typical for newly enlisted service people starting their basic training. There are no luxuries or extras here, and I easily spotted this information in the fine print of the paperwork we received along with our assignments.

Until a couple months ago, nurses have had a feminine appeal, and while the Army still expects us to look the part of a high-class, upstanding lady, we are also obliged to carry our weight now that we are official members of the US military.

"Does anyone know where the lady's room is?" Another woman asks.

"I believe I saw it down the hall through that door," someone directs her.

I place my belongings on my assigned bed, finding myself in between two women who appear to be taking in the surroundings as quietly as me. There is no point in acting shy at a time like this, so I turn to my right and hold out my hand. "I'm Elizabeth," I say, introducing myself to my neighbor's back. She spins around on her heels and returns the gesture.

"Isabel," she replies quietly. Isabel has little makeup on compared to the other women. Her skin is fair and her short, curled hair is as dark as night. Her almond-shaped blue eyes are and wide with wonder, giving her a natural look of compassion. "It's a pleasure to meet you. Where are you from?"

"Honolulu. How about you?"

"Goodness, what a place to be these past couple months, and you have come such a far way? Before the attack on Pearl Harbor, my greatest wish was to visit the islands someday. It must have been like living in paradise, especially compared to this chilly place. I have lived here in Massachusetts my entire life."

"Hawaii can be wonderful, yes. Well, until this past December, but the islands are beautiful and much like paradise. I've spent most of my life on the naval base there, but I had plenty of time in the sand and sun. I've never seen snow until today, though. It has been something I've always wanted to do, so I was quite excited for my first step into the frozen slush. But, gosh, it is much colder than I could have expected here."

"Oh dear, yes, it's even cold for those of us who lived here all our lives. This winter has been miserable so far."

Well, I suppose if I'm going to experience a New England winter, it might as well be memorable. I stroll along the outside of my cot and approach the bed on the other side. "Hi, I'm Elizabeth and that there is Isabel," I say, introducing us.

"It's a pleasure," the woman says. Her accent is thick with a rushed sound. Unlike Isabel, she has a face full of makeup, her nails painted, and jewelry that looks like it might cost more than a car. She also has dark hair, but it's pinned back and hanging below the back of her shoulder blades. "I'm Beverly from New York City — Long Island, to be specific."

"Well, that explains the accent. I've heard New Yorkers have a way with words," I say, smiling to make light of the comment. Everett told me about the few times he was in New York and how different the people acted, even different from other large cities like Los Angeles. He said the accents were strong, and the attitudes were often larger than life, but he met none other than wonderful people from the "Big Apple," as he called it.

"Oh yeah, we're always in such a big hurry that we don't have time to pronounce our R's. True story," she jests back. "Boston accents aren't much better, but I don't hear anything too strong with you, Isabel."

"Suburbia will do that to you," Isabel replies.

"I guess so. Well, at least the three of us can say we know another person here now, huh? It's nice to meet you ladies. Hopefully, we get to stick together around here, you know?" Beverly says.

"That would be nice," I agree.

As Beverly is hanging some of her street clothes, I notice an enormous diamond on her ring finger. None of us could enlist if married, so I assume she must be engaged to a man back home. "What a beautiful ring," I say.

"Oh my Gosh," Isabel follows, scurrying over to get a closer look. "That rock is huge."

Beverly inspects the ring for a long second. "I'm surprised to have this on my finger, to be honest. Johnny, my boyfriend—err —fiancé was not on board with me enlisting, but I spent years becoming a nurse and I want to see the world, you know? He's already settled down working at his father's investment company and doesn't have the motivation to seek adventure like me. I figured it's going to be now or never if I plan to spend the rest of my life with him. Honestly, I thought he was breaking things off with me before I left yesterday, but to my surprise, he popped the question. Bing, bang, boom. We're engaged to be wed, but who knows when that'll happen."

"Well, he obviously doesn't want you to forget about him while you're gone," Isabel says.

"Please, I'm sure he'll have forgotten about me within a week. All those secretaries flocking through his office building every day, he'll get bored and we all know what bored men do, right? The ring was just a way for him to make sure I didn't take up with another guy."

"I'm fortunate to have no experience with a man like this, but it looks like I might have opportunities to see how slimy some men can be," Isabel continues with a sinful wink.

The conversation brings me a sense of unease, so I turn to my suitcase and begin pulling articles of clothing out to hang up. It doesn't take me long before I'm settled and waiting for our next set of orders. I take a seat on my stiff mattress and reach over for my coat, draped over the metal frame. The silky-smooth finish of the photo paper meets my fingertips as I reach into the pocket. I pull the black-and-white image out and stare into Everett's eyes for a long moment. I'm not ready for the words on the back yet, but the smitten look of pride written across his face is exactly what I needed to see. The urge to kiss his face is strong, but I'm not ready to answer questions about him yet, so I slip the photograph into my journal I set down on top of the trunk.

I'm not sure if this is what I was expecting prior to my arrival, but I desperately need to always keep busy to avoid my thoughts going haywire. Hopefully, tomorrow will be more enlightening and allow us a chance to learn more about what we will do here in basic training.

35

JUNE 1942

SIX MONTHS, and two season changes have come and gone. From single digit temperatures with snow and ice, to days of rain and damp air, to temperatures in the mid-nineties, which is rare for June in New England, I feel like I might be acclimated for any kind of weather for wherever we end up. I can say for certain our training has prepared us for the unexpected and the inevitable. We have been pushed to the edge of our physical capabilities and filled our brains with more knowledge than I thought we could retain, but if we aren't prepared for war now, we will never be.

For a person who has never needed to plan out what happens next in life, I'm sitting with a bit of unease as I hold my focus on the foreboding look in Captain Landry's dark eyes, waiting to hear what will follow this unexpected announcement. She doesn't waver at the idea of changing directions or being in the throes of unscheduled events, but she seems unusually flustered today.

"We will leave immediately for Camp Kilmer. Once we are there, we will prepare to embark on the ship that will take us overseas." Captain Landry clasps her fingers together in front of her waist. "The number of nurses in our unit was originally higher, but because of those who didn't make it through training, we cannot meet our original quota. However, we received approval to move forward with our current resources. I don't want you ladies to walk into this situation blindly. I expect our tasks to be harder, longer, and more rigorous than anything you've encountered before now. With that said, I know what we can accomplish together."

Our unit started with over sixty nurses, but we are down to forty-one. Training proved to be more difficult for some. After years of preparing mentally for our work, the physical regimen was intense and unforgiving. There were times I didn't think I would make it through to the next day, but somehow, I persevered and put mind over matter. Giving up was not an option and now, after six months of conditioning, it's difficult to hear that we should expect more of a challenge than what we were expecting. We had no advanced warning of when we might move or deploy. Some days it felt like we were working toward an endless goal, but it was all to prepare for this moment—a moment with a road leading down a dark tunnel of unanswered questions. We don't know where we will end up following Camp Kilmer, but we are told to ignore the spinning thoughts and take the days as they come. Of all people, I should be okay with the lack of information, but I'm not. My stomach feels like it's twisting into tight knots and my heart is racing. The other women who are standing side by side in our semi-circle appear equally reluctant, but the choice is not ours to make. We have to go where we are told. That's what we signed up for.

Once dismissed, I have orders to follow before decampment, but if there was one solid piece of advice, I received in all the letters from Dad over the months; it was to keep my belongings organized and prepared to pack at a moment's notice. The time I'm allotted when it's time to move, I will want to use for tying up any loose ends.

"I heard we were being deployed to Africa," I overhear Beverly gossiping with Isabel.

"Who'd you hear that from?" Isabel responds with her typical doe-eyed look.

"Oh, you know how word gets around in the mess hall. I heard two of the boys talking over their coffee this morning."

I know better than to go by gossip. There could be multiple organizations deploying simultaneously, or we could all be going to one location, but we won't know until we are told.

After emptying the wall cabinet next to my cot, I neatly place my hygiene supplies in the appropriate spaces in my canvas duffle bag. A small stack of note paper, envelopes, stamps, and a pen is all I have left to pack. I kneel in front of my empty footlocker and rest a piece of paper on top of an envelope.

Because tomorrow cannot be a promise.

My Dearest Everett,

It's only been a couple days since I've written to you last, but I want to let you know that I'm moving to New Jersey to prepare for the next leg of my journey. I'm not sure how long I will be there or where I will go next, but I suppose that's the adventure in all of this, right?

Excitement. Everett, I'm not excited. I'm petrified, to be honest. Maybe all the years I spent declaring how unimportant our tomorrows are is coming back to haunt me. The unknown has never scared me as much as it does now. Of course, the state of the world, in its current condition, is only adding to my fears. Goodness, my intent of this letter was to let you know I am all right and trudging forward to New Jersey, not to release my troubles onto your already burdened shoulders. If I wasn't nearly out of time, I might tear up this letter and start from scratch, but I only have a few minutes left before I must report at transportation.

Everything will be fine, and I know I am more than prepared for what comes next. Like I mentioned last week, I can see muscles in my arms that I didn't know existed. Surely, that means I'm strong enough to handle whatever lies ahead. Of course, I don't quite stare at my reflection like some others do here, but the training has prepared me for a good old-fashioned arm-wrestling match. You owe me one when I see you. I'm sitting here like a fool, laughing at the words I'm writing. The other girls already think I'm a little wacky for the number of times I write you letters, but I also think they are jealous by the amount of mail I receive from the famous Everett Anderson. Besides, when I write to you, it feels almost like I'm speaking directly to your soul. I suppose that might be one good thing for all the talking I've done during our relationship. It's not completely abnormal for me to go on and on without hearing a response. At least when you write me letters, I can't interrupt you. That must be something, huh?

Thank you for making me feel better in my last few minutes here at Fort Devens. Hopefully, you are laughing at my words by this point, but that only means I've caused you to smile — the smile you said you reserved only for me.

I hope your paratroopers passed their tests this week. Of course, with you as their guide, I expect nothing less.

I miss you with all my heart, Everett.

Thinking of you always.

Love,

Lizzie

I pull out my small bottle of perfume and pump a small mist onto the paper and leave a crisp lipstick-stained kiss on the back before sealing my words into the envelope.

"Gosh, you are going to be sick of each other by the time you get to see one another again," Beverly yammers. "Is that your third letter this week?"

"So, what if it is?" I reply with a shrug. Beverly seems sour every time I am writing a letter or receiving one because Johnny has made little of an effort to respond to her love letters. She's convinced he's busy, but I worry about the heartache he might end up causing her. He doesn't seem like the most loyal man, especially after the one time he came to visit. He was enjoying the attention from the other nurses rather than his fiancée, who spent the evening pawing at him like a hungry puppy. It's not my place or any of the other girls' places to involve ourselves in her relationship, but we all feel the same about Johnny. I assumed she would have spotted someone better on base by now, but I came to find her wandering eyes are just a show. She is madly in love with Johnny and has no desire to look elsewhere.

"Now that I'm going to be near New York, I'll be able to see my Johnny again. I can't wait to call him and tell him the news later," Beverly gushes.

"How far away is Long Island from Camp Kilmer?" Isabel asks, taking a seat on my cot.

"With traffic, it might take him a couple hours, but it beats the six-hour ride it took him to visit me here. I'm sure he will be absolutely thrilled to find out how close I will be," Beverly continues.

Isabel offers me a side glance with a quick lift of her brow. I can only imagine how this will turn out for Beverly.

My bags are all set, and I peer around to see if any of the others need help with their belongings. Everyone is securing their bags or refreshing coats of lipstick except for Margaret, or "Maggie" as she goes by. She's usually the last of us to be ready, but not because she's slow. Her nerves get the best of her all too often. I walk down to her bed where she's huffing and sighing while trying to fit her hygiene products into her duffle bag.

"Here, let me help," I offer.

"I can never get this right. I must be a complete dummy," she says, pushing a fallen strand of her blonde hair off her forehead.

"Don't talk about yourself like that, Maggie. The pockets are in the same shapes as the containers, but I didn't realize this right away either. But now that you know, I bet you'll never forget."

Maggie straightens her jacket as if correcting her unsteady disposition. "Why are you so kind to me when I've done nothing to help you throughout all of our training?" She takes a hold of my elbow and twists me around to face her. "You're the only one who has been so sweet to me. I appreciate your patience with my lack of abilities."

"You are perfectly capable of all tasks, just as the rest of us are, Maggie. When you own your confidence, you will feel it too," I tell her.

I worry about her a lot, and it isn't because she shows her nerves at everyday challenges, but more for when we aren't only practicing medicine; for when we face the unimaginable horrors of war. Our jobs require a bedside manner to comfort patients, and if we are nervous nellies, it can do more harm than good for the ones we are helping. We've practiced emergency procedures until we were weak in the knees, but it's different in real-life catastrophes. The attack on Pearl was an experience I wouldn't wish on anyone, even if it gave me an advantage in knowing how to deal with severe injuries and death. I don't want to share the tragedy and misfortune I had to witness. It's unnecessary to scare the others, but there is no time to hesitate or become weak. I can only hope Maggie will find her strength in a time of need like I did. I suppose no one truly knows how tough they are until it's time to prove it to themselves.

"I certainly hope so," Maggie says, wrapping her arms around me for a hug. "I feel better knowing you don't seem nervous in the slightest bit."

* * *

A long day of travel has led us to a damp little ocean lined town. The camp looks like Fort Devens, a bit drab but brand new and still under some construction. Regardless, there is no shortage of activity.

"Lizzie, wait up." Isabel is running along to catch up. "Is it true we're only here to prepare for leaving again?"

Once the others from my barrack block at Fort Devens found out I was a military brat, the questions became endless. I will always answer everything to the best of my knowledge, but I'm not sure they understand I know as little as they do. Living life on a Naval base didn't offer me secret insights to the inner workings of how operations roll out. I believe this might be the reason Dad was always so quiet after a long day. The less he talked, the less he would have to avoid topics he couldn't discuss. Or at least, it's what I assume after the little time I've spent on this side of the Army for the last six months.

"I know just as little as you do, sweetie. We won't know anything until it happens."

"But what else would be the point of sending us to New Jersey of all places if we weren't preparing for something."

It's obvious we are preparing for a deployment, but no matter how much we find out, we will not have any in-depth details of what our mission will be. The higher-ranking nurses have explained this many times, but it seems hard for some to wrap their heads around.

"We're always preparing for something, aren't we?" I respond.

"Well, of course, but what if we aren't mentally prepared enough for whatever we're expected to do next?"

"We are," I assure her. I can't completely convince myself of this, but it's the only option we have at the moment. We have to assume we are ready for anything that happens.

"Good evening, ladies. Welcome to Camp Kilmer." A soldier with a hop in his step stops so sharply in his tracks, dust flies up around him as he removes his cap and bows toward us. He doesn't seem as nervous and stressed for time as everyone else moving around the base does. "I hope you all find the stay warm and welcoming." The man offers us a wink before continuing on his path. At the same moment, Isabel discretely snatches my gloved hand and squeezes so hard I lose feeling in the tips of my fingers.

"I assure you; the pleasure is all ours," Isabel responds, sounding giddy considering the situation we are unknowingly walking into.

Our small crowd of nurses stick together as we head toward our assigned barracks. The walk is enough time to give us an idea of how life works around here. It seems every man is on a mission to complete a task twice as fast as another guy. Everyone is in a rush to get wherever they are going, and I can't help but wonder what they know versus what we as newcomers know. My suspicion is we are here to move fast and depart even faster. Captain Landry gave us little warning before leaving Fort Devens, which tells me we are at the brink of a drastic change, an imminent attack, or an incoming threat. I don't get the feeling many of us will rest soundly tonight while we all sit and wait for our next orders.

"It is certain we need a distraction. We should go out for a night in the city," Beverly hisses in my left ear. "The tension is so thick; we need a knife to cut through it all. I'm sure you all agree we could all use a break from the mysterious mission, am I right?"

"Sure, that sounds like a swell idea." I think.

36

SEPTEMBER 1942

I'M CURLED up against the wall in the hallway of my barracks, tangled within the phone's coiled cord while waiting for an airman to put Everett on the phone. The only time the two of us can catch each other on the telephone is first thing in the morning before zero five hundred hours or just after supper.

"Doll-face." His breathy whisper sends chills up the back of my spine. I could have easily lost track of the time that has passed since we've seen each other, but I know it has been two-hundred-and-twenty-four days since I left Oahu—since I kissed his lips goodbye at the airport.

"Hi, handsome," I say, facing the wall so no one hears me.

"Finally, it's the last day of quarantine for you, huh?"

"Honest to goodness, Everett, these have been the longest ten days of my life, but I've gotten a lot of studying done, and no one else contracted meningitis. I suppose we're in the clear now."

"Good, I'm glad to hear you are all okay and safe. But what on earth are you studying now?"

"Oh, you know, just the Medical Department Soldier's Handbook for the fortieth time."

"That book is literally a pill," he jokes.

"No kidding."

"Say, Everett, I only have a minute before I have to pass the phone along. There are at least three sets of puppy dog eyes staring at my backside, waiting to call their future misses."

"I miss you," I whisper.

"I love you like crazy, doll," he shouts. Catcalls, hoots, and hollers from nearby airmen trail behind his words. They all like to get each other wound up when their girls call.

"I love you too."

"All right then, I'll talk to you soon, sweetheart."

"Everett," I stop him before he hangs up the phone.

"I'll be careful on the jumps. I promise you," he says as if it's become a routine response to his name.

"No, I know you will. It's not that. Tomorrow—I think I know what tomorrow brings."

Everett clears his throat and I hear a muffling scratch across the phone's receiver.

"Tomorrow," he says under his breath.

"I have a feeling." My words ignite a chill—stress of the unknown.

"Letters won't stop us from talking. We'll get through this. Just keep writing. Promise me, Lizzie?"

I swallow hard before responding, wishing everything ahead of us will be as simple as a promise. "Of course."

"If it isn't tomorrow, call me when you can, will you, darling?"

"Of course, silly." I try to offer a laugh, a hint that I'm not as scared as I am, but I'm sure he hears the truth.

"Stay safe, doll-face. I'll talk to you soon."

The phone dial blares in my ear and my heart pounds against the inside of my chest. Everett is only quick with goodbyes when he's upset. I've had to base his emotions off the speed of our salutations and I hate the feeling of leaving him in the same suspense I am living within, but I won't waste a chance to say goodbye out loud.

* * *

My assumptions were accurate. We received deployment orders and within hours we were ready to debark from New York Port to our next unknown destination. There are plenty of assumptions going around on where we are heading, but no one is certain. For our safety, no one will have access to further intelligence until we arrive. At the moment, everyone seems strangely calm and filled with jubilation of its own brand. Maybe it has something to do with the calmness of the sea surrounding us for as far as we can view, but none of us are blind to the fact that we are closely monitoring the vicinity for enemy submarines.

"She's at it again," Beverly moans. "Someone please make it all stop." Beverly pulls her pillow over her face and rolls over in her rack to steal a few more minutes of sleep. We should all be supporting each other in any possible way, but Beverly has been acting like an egg since the second week after we arrived in New Jersey. Johnny never came to see her and then we were quarantining because of the meningitis scares. A week later, here we are in the middle of the Atlantic.

I climb down from my rack and kneel by Maggie's side. She has been vomiting on and off daily for the last three days. Her skin has taken on a permanent shade of green and she's so weak, we can hardly get her to stand for more than a few minutes at a time. "Isabel, can you find some water?"

Isabel is out of her rack within seconds, rubbing her eyes and searching for Maggie's canteen. The ship is still pitch black because the sun hasn't hit the horizon yet and we can't use any form of lighting within the dark hours. This news did not come lightly to some members on board, but once everyone understood what could happen if an enemy spotted us at night, the questions died down and there were no further issues with complying to orders. No one could have prepared us for what to expect. However, I had already lived through many nights of darkness after the attack on Pearl. I understand the importance of staying out of sight. After the initial shock of the newly installed rules, most of us quickly adapted and have gotten proficient at feeling around for what we need at night or in the early morning hours, but it's challenging when mildly sleep deprived.

I rub Maggie's back until Isabel returns with her water and toothbrush. "Do you want me to find you some salt crackers?"

"No, thank you," Maggie croaks.

Isabel and I sit by Maggie's side, trying to comfort her in the only way we can. "I'm betting this trip won't be much longer," I tell her. It's been almost two weeks since we set sail and it's hard to know for sure, but from what I can tell with this old compass Dad gave me before I left, I'm almost certain we're heading toward Europe, which means we should dock within a couple of days.

"Am I the only one who is this sick?" Maggie asks between small sips of water.

"No, in fact, I had to hydrate four sailors yesterday after excessive spells of sickness," I say. For the most part, no one is talking about those who are incredibly seasick, but it could be much worse if the waters were choppier than they are. So far, the trip has been smooth. "Did you hear about BB last night?" Isabel asks us both, likely trying to distract Maggie from thinking about her nausea.

"No, what happened?" I ask. Nothing will come as a surprise to me with Betsy. I should have known from the initial bus ride with her that she might be too much to handle, but to be fair, I used to be the wild one in my small circle of friends. Betsy is on a whole different level of vivaciousness, though. It appears her only reason for being here is to find a man to bring home at the end of the war, but this isn't the best place to be looking for a husband, at least not now. She may have been better suited to do that in a nightclub. The last I heard, she had a notepad full of hash marks, keeping track of how many men she wooed off to a utility closet somewhere.

"Captain Landry caught her and an officer in one of the isolation wards. Last I heard, they're both in trouble on multiple accounts."

I can't say I'm surprised to hear this gossip, but a doll-dizzy officer has more to risk than Betsy does, and I find the news somewhat shocking to hear they decided an isolation ward was a good place for engaging in misconduct. "Gosh, I figured it was only a matter of time before she got caught up in more trouble than she'd be able to find her way out of. I didn't think it would happen on the ship, though."

"She's been looking for trouble since the first week of basic training when she and a private got caught, him with his pants down, while they were making whoopee in a meat-locker behind the mess hall," Isabel adds.

Her statement and reminder of that occurrence makes Maggie laugh a bit, and it's the first time we've seen her perk up since we boarded the Queen Mary.

"Who would have thought we would have so much entertainment along with this grueling lifestyle," Maggie says.

The scandalous chatter of the gossip on board the ship fills most of my letters to Everett. He isn't sure if or when he will deploy since they are still deep in training at Fort Benning in Georgia, but I've noticed he seems to have an aversion to the discussions of my impending deployment. I'm not sure if it's because he's eager to deploy or if it's because he'd prefer that I was the one still stateside. I know this though; having an ocean between us has brought with it a new sense of longing. It's Mom's words that make me think this way: "Distance is the food, stirring the hunger of love." It was something she would say whenever Dad had to go away for a bit. I couldn't understand why she wasn't in a mess of tears like I was when he left, but now I realize it was because she would only allow herself to think about how happy she would be upon his return. To look at the distance between Everett and I as a way of making our love even stronger is better than focusing on the constant ache in my chest.

Just as we seem to get Maggie settled into a place of comfort, a growing echo of sirens bounces off the metal walls, startling all of us up to our feet. Within seconds, we're in our uniforms, our boots tied, and we are piling into the corridor to reach our assigned locations to prepare for an incoming air raid. As it has each day since we've been onboard, my heart sinks to the darkest cavern of my chest as I recall the sounds, the sights, smells and emotions of the attack on Pearl. This may be just another drill, or it may be the real thing. Either way, we must act and react, face the fear of what might come our way. As nurses, our job is to prepare for the worst and hope for the best. For safety reasons, the nurses' sleeping quarters are on the bottom of the ship, but there are sets of stairs that lead us up to the hospital wards.

The darkness of each corridor, though, has its own dangers

because of the obstacles and barriers impeding us from finding our way around without getting hurt. I have several cuts and contusions from the middle of the night drills. Minutes pass before the sirens become a low ringing hum, informing us that our hearts can cease to pound for the moment because this is just another drill.

By the time we return to our quarters, the sun has risen enough to allow a scant amount of light to brighten the upper decks. This means we can now use whatever sources of lighting we have below deck. After being awake for hours, I'm out of sorts as I try to clear my head of the thoughts of what could have happened overnight.

"What's that?" Beverly says as she makes her way back toward her rack.

"What's what?" I question.

"That necklace. I've never seen you wearing it before. Did one of the nice anchor-crankers give it to you?" Beverly waggles her eyebrows at me, but I refrain from reacting to her teasing remarks. She likes to get a rise out of me, and the others, but I refuse to let her think she's accomplishing whatever it is she's trying to do.

I slip my necklace back beneath my collar and ignore her question. By the look on her face, I can see she isn't about to let the questions go without answers. She takes the few steps between us and corners me between the wall and the rounded hatch. When she reaches toward me, I slap her hand away. "Do you mind?" I ask.

"What are you hiding, Lizzie?" She always puts emphasis on the last part of my name, as if she's accusing me of something.

"I'm not hiding anything. What does it matter to you?" My words will do nothing but start an argument with Miss New York, who cannot let anything go.

"Leave her alone," Isabel calls out as she's unlacing her boots.

"I saw what it was. It doesn't matter," Beverly says.

"So what?" I reply.

"Are you hoping to get us all locked up or something?"

"What in the world are you talking about?" Isabel states, walking toward us.

"Your closest gal pal here is a Jew. A proud one at that, it seems. How did I not realize this before? Your last name is a dead giveaway. Your pretty blonde curls make for a good distraction, I guess."

I'm in a state of shock while digesting each one of Beverly's words. I wasn't hiding my faith, but it hadn't been brought up in any conversation we've had.

"What is wrong with you?" I ask.

I know what is happening in Europe and I plan to be more careful with my necklace if we are in a dangerous area, but I'm on board with all Americans now, and one of them is turning on me as if it's a natural reaction to a person of the Jewish faith.

"Me?" She squawks, sounding flabbergasted at my question.

"We're probably three-quarters of our way to Europe, where Jews are being locked up and killed. And here you are, strutting around with that necklace on as we enter whatever enemy territory we're heading into?"

"Stop it right now," Maggie says from the edge of her rack. "Why would you say such a horrible thing?"

"Oh please, you're more of a flight risk than Lizzie with your nervous nelly routine. Do any of you understand what we're about to walk into?"

I'm stuck on Beverly's initial comments rather than what she's still gabbing about.

"Are you really Jewish?" Diane, another nurse asks.

"Yes, it's not quite the disease you're making it sound like though."

I never assumed Dad's warnings weren't true, but I hoped these women I've spent the last six months with, who I thought were my friends, weren't the type to hold judgment based on a person's beliefs. Nurses should be kind to all without prejudice, and I'm appalled at the ensuing topic.

"Well, I didn't say it was," Diane says. "But Beverly has a point. What if we're around the Germans who are trying to exile all the Jews from Europe? We could all end up in danger, Elizabeth."

My pulse is buzzing within my ears, and my cheeks feel like

they are on fire. "I will make sure no one else finds out I am a Jewish woman. However, I will not be apologizing for who I am."

Maggie and Isabel are silent, but it seems like they are both filled with a sense of disbelief and I don't know if it's because I'm Jewish or due to what Beverley and Diane just said.

"Honestly, I can't believe the military is allowing you to be a part of this deployment," Beverly continues. "I find your decision to be here very selfish, Elizabeth."

I'm having trouble pulling in enough air to continue this discussion. Beverly hasn't been the kindest of our group, but I didn't have her pinpointed as an antisemitic person. As much as I want to tell her I have worked just as hard as she has and been through unthinkable situations before arriving here on this ship, it won't matter to someone as shallow as she.

I corral my belongings and leave the quarters with my tongue stuck to the roof of my mouth. I no longer feel fear for the moment, just anger and resentment, but I can't figure out if there is any validity behind her calling me a risk to the others.

MONTHS WENT by when many of us thought we were waiting like sitting ducks, wondering why we continue to move around the United Kingdom, often between England and Scotland. We have been short on personnel since arriving here almost a year ago, but until recently we were doing little to aid in the efforts of the war. We had more downtime than expected, and the free moments left our minds to wander and our hearts yearning for home. To make matters worse, the weather here in England is neither here nor there. It's not frigid like in Boston, but the sky is gloomy and gray most of the time and it leaks like a broken faucet most days. With a lack of sunshine, I'm certain we are all deficient in vitamin D. It's not truly the weather that has me down, though. I seem to have lost my spirit over these last few months. I haven't heard from Everett in over two months. The last letter he wrote to me mentioned there could be a gap in communication for a while because of his upcoming mission, but I don't have the faintest idea where in this world he is or if he's even all right.

Daily casualties among US airmen trickle in. The predominance of injuries is due to the explosions, but most of our men have been lucky as there have been few deaths. Still, each time I see the Army Air Corps uniform, my insides collapse as if the bones in my body are weaker than a piece of wet paper. I inspect each patient for familiar eyes, but none have come close to the only ones I want to see.

I find myself in a cycle of repetition in triage most days. I'm the first to unwrap initial coats of dressing, revealing the level of severity of each injury. Depending on the location of the wound, and whether we can loosen a tourniquet without the patient hemorrhaging, determines where he will go next. We take on whatever tasks we can to treat in this initial location as this frees up the operating rooms and long-term care beds.

The biggest difference between working in an evacuation hospital and the naval hospital is our goal of transporting men out as fast as possible, often hoping we've made the right decision. The level of trust left on our shoulders to think quickly and choose wisely makes it hard to sleep some nights.

"Lizzie, could you check on Benjamin? I cannot get the bleeding to stop and the tourniquet is as tight as I can make it. I can help with Frank's sutures if you wouldn't mind," Isabel asks. Her words pull me out of another dark haze of repetition while checking for infection, fevers, and other previously undisclosed injuries. Frank arrived a couple hours ago with a laceration to his forefinger.

"Of course," I tell her. "I've just finished checking for nerve damage. It doesn't appear that the shrapnel cut deep enough to cause more than a superficial laceration. He needs about fifteen stitches."

I place my hand on Frank's pale face, wondering why some of these soldiers have such boyish features when they are fighting as men. "Isabel is going to fix you right up and we'll get you out of here as soon as possible." I offer my typical calming smile and Frank grabs my elbow with his good hand.

"Miss, I would like to thank you for taking care of me."

"Of course, it's my pleasure." I lean away from his hand to continue toward Benjamin, but Frank's hand tightens and won't release me.

"I'm sorry to bother you and sound like a stuttering fool, but I don't want to miss the opportunity to ask you if you'd like to have dinner with me tonight or some other night this week. We'll be in town for a bit, and it sure can feel lonely around here. You remind me of home, Miss."

His eyes widen, much like a child waiting to find out what prize they won at a fair.

"Frank, it's awfully kind of you to ask, but I'm afraid I can't join you for dinner."

"Oh, I beg your pardon, Miss. I didn't mean to make such an assumption. I should have asked if you are taken before assuming you would jump at such a forward offer." Truthfully, I'm not sure if I'm taken, left behind, or forgotten about.

"There's no need for regret, sweetheart. I'm not so patiently waiting to hear from the one I'm taken by. He's also in the Army Air Corps, but I don't believe he is part of your unit."

"You don't say," Frank continues. A pink color fills in the white areas of his cheeks as if I offered him a bit of relief. "What's his name, if you don't mind me asking?"

I've learned that men do not have the same reaction when hearing Everett's name, not like the response I get when telling one of the other nurses. "Lieutenant Everett Anderson is his name."

Frank stares through me for a long moment, as if he's going through a catalog of names in his head. "I'm afraid I don't know of him, but I have heard some other units from the states are seeing far more than we are, but there are also some who aren't seeing much at all. Miss, I'll pray for you and him. All we can do is hope he isn't on the front lines."

"How kind of you." Frank releases his grip and I make eyes at Isabel—a look the two of us share when we run into an overly eager homesick soldier or airman. Isabel is free as a bird, but I know what makes her blush, and I find it mildly amusing that as sweet as she is, it's the boys with the dirty mouths that make her giggle. I'm afraid Frank might remind her more of the kid brother she left back home.

As I move over to Benjamin, I notice a particular look in his eyes, a cold, expressionless stare toward the ceiling. "How long has Benjamin been like this?" I call over to Isabel.

"Like what?" she responds.

"Unresponsive."

"I was talking to him just a minute ago," she says, turning back toward Frank.

"Benjamin," I say sternly, looking for a reaction. His eyes don't blink and there is no change in the rhythm of the pulsating artery on the side of his neck.

"Benjamin, if you can hear me, I need you to blink or say something, darling." Again, there's nothing. He's in shock. I carefully unwrap the soaked tourniquet, finding the bleeding to be much heavier than what I'd assumed it would be. I grab a clean roll of dressing and re-wrap the wound while applying pressure on the brachial artery on the inside of his bicep. The wrap was too low before and wasn't offering enough compression. He's lost a lot of blood between the time he arrived and now. His lips have a blue tint, and I'm not comfortable with the level of paleness.

"We need blood, Isabel. Where is Nancy? Can you see if she's in the next unit?"

"A positive, correct?" Isabel responds.

"Yes, Ma'am, I confirm while scanning down the length of Benjamin's intake paper."

"What's the matter with Benny?" Frank calls over. "He's not dying or anything, is he?"

"You don't need to worry," I respond. "We just need to replace the blood he lost. He'll be fine." I've gotten good at lying so easily with a complacent smile on my face. I'm certainly not God and will never know who could walk out of here and who will leave beneath a sheet. The information we receive upon intake is never enough to make assumptions or predict an outcome.

Nancy and Isabel are hustling when they return with two pint bags.

"Let me set this up for you so you can clean up," Nancy offers.

I'm covered in Benjamin's blood, which has become a common occurrence in our unit the past week with the airmen under attack by the Germans. I think the days of me not having enough to keep my mind occupied are over.

I slowly release the pressure on his artery, hoping not to feel the warmth of another rush of blood. The unease of knowing if what I did was enough, never subsides. We're all silent for the long few seconds I wait with my hands an inch from his arm.

"You did well, Lieutenant Salzberg," Nancy says. She's newer to our unit, brought over to replace a few of our nurses who left for another location. She's been a nurse for about fifteen years, but only recently completed her basic training after enlisting. It feels unusual to own any semblance of authority over someone who has more experience than me, but we all start at the same place in the Army—the bottom. However, I suspect everyone will view her as a motherly figure around here in no time. She has quickly taken a liking to the rest of us and dotes on us as if we're her daughters when we aren't working. It's been nice having her with us these last couple of weeks.

I watch in awe as Nancy seamlessly sets up the bag of blood while holding a steady conversation with Benjamin, even though he isn't alert. Maybe someday I won't be faking my calmness, or I'll become as good as she is at keeping that secret to myself.

"Look at that, those perky lips of yours are already turning a delightful shade of pink again. I believe you are going to be just fine, Corporal."

"You're a natural," I tell Nancy.

"And you," she says, turning around to place her hands on her hips. "Go clean up. Then I want to hear about the reason for those tired bags beneath your gorgeous eyes." I roll my "gorgeous" eyes at her and head across the room toward the sink.

Either I'm taking too long to scrub my hands or Nancy is more concerned than she lets on.

"Lizzie, what's going on? You don't look right today." She isn't talking to me as a comrade anymore, just as the older, wiser figure many of us desperately need. We've gotten good at calling each other by rank when appropriate and by name when there's a minute to squeeze in a personal conversation.

"Oh, I'm just fine," I say, spewing yet another lie.

"I've only known you less than two weeks, but you look tired. Are you feeling all right?"

"It's the exhaustion, I'm sure. I keep waking up at zero three hundred hours, thinking it's time to get moving. My mental alarm clock is out of whack."

A small smile perks to one side of Nancy's lips. "I have a daughter who is about five years older than you, and do you know I got so good at detecting what her mood changes meant, I sometimes knew what was going on before she did?"

Mom was like that with me. She would always tell me that my emotions were so colorful anyone could see them from miles away. Yet, I do what I can to hide every emotion running through my head, knowing personal struggles do not have a place here in the trenches of war.

"She sounds like a lucky daughter to have you for a mom," I say.

"Was," Nancy says, taking my breath away. "She got sick, and we thought it was influenza, but it turned out she had a large tumor no one knew about. By the time we found out what was going on, it was too late. We lost her a few weeks after she got sick. Some nurse I am, huh?"

"You can't blame yourself," I scold her. I shouldn't be quick to reprimand when I spent years blaming myself from Mom's death, and there was no truth to the reasons I had, but it allowed me to be angry at myself rather than deal with the grief. "I understand, Nancy. My mom died seven years ago. Sometimes it feels better to take the blame."

Nancy pulls in a sharp breath and straightens her shoulders. "I think I know why we are both here, Lizzie."

"Me too."

"I also think you look tired because you haven't heard from Everett, and I can only assume you were listening to the radio with the others this morning as news broke about allies stepping into Italy."

It's as if she took the thoughts directly from my mind and read them like a type-written story.

"He isn't here. At least I don't think he is, but something doesn't feel right. After the attack on Pearl, I didn't know where he was for a day. It felt like a month, though. But now, not hearing from him for two months is killing me. I'm not sure how much more my heart can take, Nancy."

Nancy wraps her hand around my chin and lifts my face to meet her eyes. Her short coppery hair and matching bright eyes offer so much warmth. "You are more than strong enough to keep going, and your strength is likely keeping him safe. Let's imagine that he is doing what he loves; flying through the clouds and sending you dozens of letters that just aren't moving nearly as fast as he is. The likelihood of that situation is far more believable than the worst-case scenario."

My face fills with warmth and my throat tightens while I take in the words I desperately needed to hear, but the moment is over as quickly as it began when I spot movement over Nancy's shoulder. Benjamin is squirming and groaning with pain.

"He needs morphine. Let's make him more comfortable by reducing the pain," I tell Nancy while racing back to Benjamin's bedside.

38

CURRENT DAY – OCTOBER 2018

THIS DAY HAS GONE by in a flash, just as the rest. The sun rises and sets again and again. But when the sun dips below the horizon, I will say goodnight to my life until tomorrow because it's too hard on my old eyes to see in the dark.

"Sweetheart, everyone is here. Can I help you downstairs?" Keiki asks.

I glance down to my wrist where my watch should be, but I only find smudged, brown age spots splattered across my pale skin. "Keiki, shouldn't you be off duty now? Your family must miss you, being gone all day."

Keiki takes my hand and helps me up from my porch seat. "My family is downstairs," she explains.

I look up into her dark enchanting eyes, finding a reciprocating look of wonder. "What a wonderful idea—to invite your family over, too. Well, I should have thought of that. The more the merrier, of course."

Keiki presses her lips together into a tight-lipped smile. "Come on, sweetheart."

"We should eat dinner out on the terrace. It's a beautiful night," I continue while following her lead.

"We are eating out on the terrace. This is the lanai to your bedroom."

I feel a tightness tug at the skin on my forehead. What in the world is she talking about? I've been having family dinners out on that terrace for more than half of my life. I glance over my shoulder toward the open glass doors. Maybe she's confused.

When we arrive at the bottom of the open stairwell, I spot a gathering on the other side of the kitchen.

"The terrace," Keiki says, pointing toward the crowd.

I hate when my mind feels like it has been spinning in dizzying circles for hours. It's hard to question myself—whether my thoughts are accurate or incoherent. It's times like this when I prefer to remain quiet and unresponsive to whatever I'm questioning.

"Here she is! Mom, we thought you were going to make us eat without you tonight."

"Lewis?" I call out. "I haven't seen you in so long. Where have you been?"

He walks toward me with concern edging fine lines into his aging features. He takes my hand from Keiki and pulls me along but stops before stepping outside.

"Mom, look at me."

"Why do you keep calling me Mom? Is this another prank you and James are pulling on me? You know I don't enjoy your wild jokes very much."

"It's me, Carter, your son."

I lift my hand to touch his face, trying to understand what he's saying.

"Mom, is everything okay?" The voice comes from behind us, from outside.

"Leah, she needs a minute," Lewis—or Carter says.

"Makena, why is he calling you Leah?" Is everyone playing games with me tonight?

"Mom, Makena is my daughter, with Cliff, your son-in-law. And Carter is here with Julia, your daughter-in-law, with their three sons."

"What on earth—" I step forward, taking a closer look outside at what must be two dozen people. "Who are all these people here? I'm unprepared for such a large festivity." I run my fingers through my hair that I didn't tend to today and I peer down at the night gown I've been resting in most of the afternoon.

"We're your family, every one of us. You have two married children, four grandchildren and their spouses, and five great-grandchildren ... so far. Look what you've done."

I scan every face, feeling a familiar warmth in my chest, but my thoughts are scattered. "I'm trying to do the numbers in my head, which never fares well for me, but there are over seventeen of you out there," I say.

"No one can say she isn't still sharp as a tack with numbers," Carter jests.

He sounds so much like Lewis, it's uncanny.

"There are more than seventeen out there. James's family is here too. He had two wonderful daughters, both are married, two grandchildren who have also married, and one great-granddaughter, if you can believe it."

"If I wasn't losing my mind, I still wouldn't be able to keep up with you right now. Exactly, how big is our family?"

"Pretty big," Leah says with Makena's matching smile.

"Hi Gran," Makena walks in, confirming she and her mother are in fact two different people who look almost identical. They look like me, or the way I once looked. Makena places a kiss on my cheek. "I'm so sorry for Daniel taking so much of your time today. He's fascinated by your story about the war, but I know you don't like to talk about it much. I told him to go easy on you, though he said you were happy to keep talking."

I don't recall a time when I wasn't happy to share my stories from the war. "Of course, darling. It was my pleasure. Daniel is such a wonderful man. I'm so glad you have met a nice man to date."

"Oh—" Makena chirps, but Leah nudges her as if I don't see their interaction.

"What about Lewis? Where is his family?"

"But, Gran," Makena tries to respond.

"Makena, go outside and find Daniel, please," Leah tells her daughter.

Leah takes my right hand and Carter takes my left and walks me out through a break in the crowd of my family members who are all looking at me as if it's the first time they are seeing me in this light. The feeling is mutual. "Lewis had a wonderful partner in life, Mom. You adored Uncle Theo. They didn't have children, but they joined the Peace Corps and traveled near and far to tend to starving families and environmental crises. They did so much good in the world and gave many people better lives."

Some of Leah's explanation rings a bell, but the memories are vague, and the name Theo sounds familiar, but I can't picture his face. "That sounds like your uncle. All he wanted was happiness for others. I spent a long time thinking I was the one who needed to follow in my mother's footsteps, but he was right there, doing the very same thing in his own way, wasn't he?"

"He was an incredible man and uncle, Mom. You were so very proud of him."

"I still am," I tell Leah. "He's gone, though?"

Leah wraps her arm around my shoulders. "James and Lewis passed away from old age just a few years ago, both within months of each other."

"And your grandfather? My father." I know it's impossible for him to still be around, but I can't remember losing him.

"Grandpa passed away at the age of a hundred-and-two. He was too stubborn to let go. He said to us: 'I will decide when it's my time, and I'm not ready yet,' but you told him he was making your mom wait an awful long time," Leah says with a giggle. "He still hung on for several months but went in his sleep that summer."

I turn to look at Leah, wishing I could see the memories within her eyes. "My head is so empty. I'm missing so much, sweetie."

"It's all there, Mom," Carter says. "It's just a lot of memories to keep track of."

"It sure is," I say, glancing back out toward the crowded table.

Keiki is setting dishes down on the table with the help of who I assume to be her husband, and there are children fleeing around with the most joyful smiles and giggles.

"How is my favorite great aunt?" The man helping Keiki rushes to my side and offers me a perfect string necklace of cherry red hibiscus flowers.

"She's your only great-aunt, you goof," Leah corrects him.

"Brandon, stop causing problems over there," Keiki calls out.

"Yes, darling," Brandon responds.

"Keiki is my housekeeper. I don't understand," I say through an unclear mutter.

Brandon lets out a boisterous laugh. "Keiki is James's granddaughter. She's a nurse and stays here to help you throughout the day."

"That's nonsense," I shout. "Why on earth would my great-niece ..." I pause, wondering if I'm correct in calling her that or if I'm still confused.

"Yes, your great-niece," Brandon says.

"Why would she be spending her prime years taking care of an old bat like me?"

Keiki interrupts with her most comforting smile. "Sweetheart, your family loves you so much that everyone has pitched in to pay the worth of my nursing salary so I can be a familiar comfort to you every day. None of us could fathom the idea of having a stranger in this house when you have so many of us. This family is unbreakable, and we all do what we can for each other no matter how much we might argue sometimes," she says, elbowing Brandon in the ribs.

My heart feels so full, yet, so empty at the same time. I don't recognize most of everyone here. Keiki, Makena, Leah, and I suppose Carter, but only because he looks like Lewis—they are all familiar, but I don't understand why everyone else looks like a stranger to me. They must have all been here before, but I don't remember any of them.

"Leah, where are James and Lewis? Why didn't they come to the party? And your father? Is he not home from work yet? It's late."

I'm not sure what I said to make everyone become so quiet at the same moment, but the sound of crickets fills the salty air.

"We're all here to celebrate Dad's birthday," Carter says.

A heaviness fills my chest while I conjure my next question. "Is it a surprise party?"

"Mom—" Leah says.

This is my world now; overflowing with empty space and questions with no answers.

39

MARCH 1944

"GOODNESS GRACIOUS," Nancy says, switching the power off on the radio as she walks by our nurses' station. "It's no wonder you have nightmares every night."

"We have to stay informed of what is happening. We'd be foolish to turn a blind eye to it all," I tell her.

"It won't change anything in this hospital, Lizzie."

"London was already attacked once. There's no saying it won't happen again," I argue. Nancy dips her hands into the deep pockets of her trench coat as if she's waiting for me to say more before responding. "Well, it's true, isn't it?"

"You, my dear, listen to the radio for updates about the Army Air Corps. There's nothing you are going to hear that will offer you peace of mind. Wherever your Everett is, the information is probably highly classified." We've had the same conversation so many times over the last eight months, and I have tried my best to shut the thoughts off but being here in London is a constant reminder of the nagging question that haunts me. "You don't know this for sure," I tell Nancy.

"Your father has said so too in his letters. You should take some comfort in his words. I'm sure he would know if something happened to Everett.

"I'm not sure what to believe anymore." I shuffle a pile of

records from our current patients and click the stack together on the countertop.

Nancy retrieves a paper bag from her pocket and places it down in front of me. "Maybe this will help."

The tattered and torn tea-brown bag looks older than me. "What is this?"

"It's a stack of mail that arrived just before I was leaving our quarters. It all came together enclosed like it is, but it's addressed to you from another unit."

I trace my fingertips along the soft touch of the worn paper, feeling a quiver move through my nerves. I carefully open the bag and retrieve the stack of letters, careful not to catch a corner on the weak seam of the bag. My hand trembles as I read my name written in black ink. "It's his handwriting," I mutter, feeling unable to take in a full breath.

I remove the twine wound around the pile and thumb through the envelopes, finding the dates in order from the most recent one being from this New Year's Day all the way back to last April. I couldn't figure out how almost a year has passed since I've heard from him, but his letters are all here. Even through all my doubts, questions, and worries, I continued to write to him. There were days I thought I might have been mailing letters to a ghost. For all I know, it could be true since the last letter is from January, three months ago.

I start with the most recent letter and hold it up to my nose, hoping to inhale a familiar a scent, but all I smell is paper and ink. The flap parts and I pull the yellow piece of notepaper out. My thoughts on what might be written inside the folds initiate a sense of panic, stiffening every muscle in my body.

"Nurse, pardon me," a patient hollers for me from behind.

"I'll help him. Take your time and read what you need to," Nancy says, placing her hand on my shoulder as I ease into the seat of the wooden folding chair.

I feel like my fingers are coated with grease as I try to part the folds. With a deep breath, I close my eyes and straighten out the full length of the paper.

My Sweet Lizzie,

It's been so long since I've heard your angelic voice, and longer since I've read your poetic words. There's been a rumor about a hold up in the mail because of a block in communications. I'm not sure if that's why I haven't heard from you, but I hope you are receiving my letters at the very least.

I've been unimaginably busy these last few weeks. There has been little time for sleep or any other extra-curricular activities some other units often get to take part in. I wish I could tell you precisely where I am, but they have prohibited us from disclosing those details. All I know is, I pray you are somewhere safe and not seeing the same appalling sights I've witnessed. I couldn't have thought anything would dull the reminders of what happened during the attack on Pearl, but I was wrong.

All I can do is tell myself you are okay, but it's not enough, Lizzie. We haven't heard many details of casualties among the Nurse Corps, and I hope it's because you are safe. Each day brings the shock of unspeakable horrors, and I wonder how much longer this war can continue.

Last week, I was in a small village with quaint family homes settled above blocks of shops. There were so many colors and rich artwork on every corner. I couldn't help but think how much you would love being there, if it was a safe place to be, of course. It's maddening that this war is the cause of destruction to so much beauty. I try my best to see through the smoke and debris, but some days are harder than others. I'm sure you are experiencing much of the same wherever you are.

As I've said in all my other letters, my heart aches when I sit down for a moment with a piece of paper and pen. You feel so far away and then I stare up at the sky and I find a hint of warmth. I tell myself you are looking at the same clouds I am, just like we promised to do. The days when the sky is clear and blue, I wonder if you're somewhere closer without the clouds separating us. I'll stare at the sun for a few seconds and when I look away, I can see your face looking down at me. Then I realize I might have lost my mind at some point throughout this past year.

I wish I had something more insightful to say, but I am missing you more than I have ever missed a thing in my entire life. I didn't know such a pain existed, but in my heart, I know it's a battle we have to fight before we can find the ending we want.

Anyway, I love you, doll-face.

Soon. It must be soon that we will see each other again.

Always and forever,
E—

The letter falls from my loose grip and drifts like a feather down to the counter. Three months have passed since this letter. He's seeing far worse than we are here, and that's the only detail given about his location. I don't understand why he hasn't received my letters, and there's no way to know if it's the same reason there isn't one dated from within the last few months. Dad's updates in his letters to me could be outdated. By the time I find out there is no recorded listing of casualties for his unit, it's at least two weeks later than when the numbers came in.

I'm not sure I feel any better than I did twenty minutes ago. Knowing he was still alive and well in January doesn't offer me comfort aside from learning he hadn't stopped writing, and he still loved when he put the heartfelt words on paper. Deep down, I couldn't see him forgetting about me, but when the mind has too many avenues to travel, the roads can end traveling down a dark path.

Nancy returns to my side with a wild look of wonder floating through her glistening bronze eyes. "Is everything okay?"

I shrug and lean my chin into my hand, allowing my elbow to slide across the counter. "It was in January, but who knows if everything is fine now."

Nancy releases a heavy sigh and places her hand across her chest. "Oh, sweetie, you went so long without a word. I don't think you should assume the worst. You shouldn't read these letters while staring at the date marked on top. The words were written by Everett at just a moment in time. Hearing his voice within your mind is what matters."

I press a small smile into the corner of my lips, wishing I could accept what she's saying, but my emotions are becoming weaker by the day, and at a time when I should be finding a new sense of strength each morning. I'm failing myself and my conviction to conquer this undertaking. "Thank you for your kind advice. I appreciate your uplifting thoughts," I tell Nancy.

She glances down at her wristwatch and back up at me. "There are only a couple more hours until your shift is over. I heard there is an event tonight. That sounds like a delightful break for you girls," Nancy says, pressing her lips into a tight line. I know she must work all night, and I I wonder if she was hoping to join us.

"Would you like to go? I don't mind working your shift," I offer in case that's what she was hinting at. Though Nancy hasn't gotten excited for a USO event like the other girls, maybe she needs to cut loose a bit too.

"Oh gosh, no, I am far too old for those events, but thank you for the offer. Plus, you work more hours than anyone else. You deserve a night out."

"They're certainly entertaining," I tell her. I don't see how everyone can shut off the troubles we've seen and lock it away during a night of entertainment. It seems I'm unable to mask the truth, even for a few hours. "Even more so if you're the one watching all the others go bananas."

"There is nothing wrong with taking it all in," Nancy insists. "We will take our laughs from wherever we can get it, right?"

She sure has a good point on that. I've almost forgotten what it feels like to laugh.

40

MARCH 1944

I FEEL foolish sitting on the train that's taking us to the location where the event is taking place. The other girls are dreaming about this perfect evening, fantasizing their wildest dreams playing out. I'm not sure I can think of a dream worthy enough of imagining, aside from the obvious, but I am also a person who keeps my focus where it should be.

Beverly nudges my knee with her toe. I glance up from the sight of my intertwined leather-clad fingers, wondering why she would be nudging me. My sight falls to her deep shade of red lipstick, and the pucker of her mouth. Her dark lined eyes narrow in on me and it's clear she has a question.

"What's the matter with you now? Why can't you smile anymore?"

I shake my head, wishing to say much more than what I will respond with. "What is there to smile about, Beverly?"

Her mouth falls ajar as if I just shared the best gossip she's heard this week. "You're a crack up, you know that? Sweetheart, you need to find yourself a doll-dizzy fella who would love to put a grin on that face of yours. It will fix all your problems, I promise you."

Everything Beverly says is rubbish, and I want to call her out on this bluff. I could point out the fact that she has been giving other men inappropriate attention when she still has

Johnny at home. He may not be sitting around waiting for the
day she comes home, or worse, he might be doing the same
thing she is, but I don't see the point in continuing a
relationship if neither person is being faithful. Beverly has made
it clear from the beginning that we will never see eye-to-eye on
matters of the heart. I've just come to accept her ignorance.
"While that sounds like a swell time, I'm not in need of a
gentleman's company right now, but I appreciate your
concern."

Beverly holds her gloved hands up and shifts her thin brows
to the side. "My apologies," she says. "Well, you look nice tonight
—very European chic, and I don't mean Eastern European—just,
you know, fashionable." Her comments can have many meanings,
but I decide to assume the best case to avoid confrontation.
Sometimes, I feel as though she pushes me to react, though. Her
cat-like gaze scans down the length of my face, settling on the
base of my neck where the chain of my necklace meets my
collarbone.

"How nice of you to say," I reply, shifting my attention to the
empty sweat between Maggie and Isabel.

"So, did you read any of the other letters yet?" Maggie asks.
Her eyes hold a sense of child-like wonder, wide with a glow of
fantastical hope. She even has her gloved hands cupped over her
heart—the true definition of a hopeless romantic waiting for
Prince Charming to show up on a white horse and whisk her
away. So far, she hasn't come across any of these fairytale men
while we were in London, which disappoints her since she thinks
we were in the land of love.

"You're savoring each one, aren't you?" Isabel asks with a
giggle. "I would probably do the same."

"I read a couple, but they were short and just sweet reminders
of times we shared before I left for the East coast."

"Say, there's a smile," Isabel coos, pursing her lips. "I'm so
glad you heard from your guy. It's the little things right now, I
understand."

"Meow, Meow, Miss popularity. You heard from that nice
boy? How come no one told me?" Beverly asks, smoothing her
fingers along the end of her scarf.

"When have you ever pretended to care?" Isabel responds with a scoffing chuckle before turning back toward me.

"Of course I care. I think we all know how badly Lizzie needs to lighten up. Am I right?" She mutters the last of her words beneath her breath, hoping we hear her but likely trying to avoid a response.

Maggie and Isabel shake their heads at Beverly while I break away from the conversation to stare out the window into the dark, foggy sky.

* * *

The masses of soldiers, sailors, and Marines cram into this dim-lit, dank space underground. Chatter from so many people at once sounds like the hum of a car's engine, growing louder the closer we get to the main function room. The moment we walk in, gawking eyes from every direction make me feel like a forbidden fruit these men have been kept from for so long. Any fellow who hasn't had the need for medical care has had little or no interaction with us women. However, the American troops are fighting for the attention of the lovely British soldiers. The nurses are quite taken by the accents. Of course, none of these men will sit back and allow the British men to steal what they might feel is theirs, so the jealousy has not gone unnoticed as the number of local British women grow at each of these events. At least, it's entertaining to watch, which is what I plan to do once I find an empty seat.

"Come dance with us, Lizzie," Isabel pleads, grabbing Maggie and me by the hands to pull us in the opposite direction from where I want to go. It's no secret she's ready to have the time of her life tonight, decked out in a black A-line skirt and her fitted, cherry-red button-down blouse. As a graduate of Wesley College, Isabel seems to have a sweet spot for mixers, a dance floor, and some good big band swing music. She's gushed about the many dances she attended while living the collegiate life. She was part of the swing dancing club too and even has trophies to show for her winnings.

"Maybe in a bit," I say, pulling my hands from hers. I do not have the same type of confidence on the dance floor. I didn't attend those types of events in Oahu.

With disappointment lacing the girls' eyes, they blow me a kiss and follow Beverly toward the excited men waving them over.

It isn't long before there's a host on stage, thanking us for continuing our civic duties. "We have a couple special guests for you tonight who want to show their appreciation for everything you are doing on behalf of the United States." The host is an older man with a sharp tan and contrasting white hair that shines beneath the hanging lights. He's in a pricey suit and his teeth are brighter than the napkins on the table next to me. Another gentleman runs out onto the risers and whispers something into the host's ear. "Well, no kidding. Who would have known?" No one knows what the man is talking about since he's only responding to the whisper into the microphone, but I suppose it's part of the teasing gig while we wait to see who is coming out to entertain us tonight.

There is a bit of commotion out in front of the platform where the host is waving someone onto the platform. These boys will get a kick out of just about anything these events stir up. A crowd of sailors shoves a man up on to the high riser, coming face to face with the host.

"Holy moly, it's really you, huh?" The host has the crowd chanting with pleas to find out who the mystery person is. The crowd is hooting and cheering as if Perry Como just showed up. "Ladies and Gentlemen, it is my great honor and dare I say, shocking revelation, to introduce you to none other than one of Hollywood's finest picture people, Everett Anderson. Excuse me, Lieutenant Everett Anderson."

My hands fly up to my chest as I clutch at the fabric of my blouse. They must be playing a joke on the crowd. There's a light blaring over the man's head, but I can't imagine Everett would be here in Edinburgh. Surely, we would have found out we were in the same location by now. The lights swivel around, and my view becomes crystal clear as I spot the man I love, alive and standing in one piece. He's staring out into the crowd as if the stage is unfamiliar to him when we all know it not to be the case.

"Sorry for the disappointment, folks, but I'm not the actual entertainment here tonight, but my buddies wanted to see me squirm under a spotlight before you find out who the true entertainer is." Everett is blushing and seems embarrassed to be up on stage, and yet, here I am, frozen to my seat. The sound of whistles and hoots from the ladies here grow into a ferocious call toward Everett, but rather than accept the attention, he spins around on his heels and offers to shake the host's hand. "I'll let you get back to your introductions now," Everett says.

I stand from my seat as if my body is floating above me and I take long strides toward the center of the room. As Everett is about to step off the platform, I call out to him. "Everett!" I realize my voice likely sounds like every other woman's voice in this place tonight, and he hasn't heard me speak in so long. I would understand if he didn't stop to see who is calling for him. Plus, there are so many arms reaching out as he jumps down from the platform.

I'm not sure if he even heard me, but I continue pushing my way through the crowd, feeling like it's been forever since I laid eyes on the man I love. The men in the front rows are all so tall and it's hard to see much from where I am, but it helps when a small path opens between two sections of people.

My heart quakes so hard I feel like I need to press my hands against my chest. Am I dreaming? He's more beautiful than I even remember. With far more muscles than he had and a harder look to the shape of his face, he looks like a matured version of the man I can vividly recall every detail of.

"Lizzie." I don't know if he is speaking my name out loud or if he's mouthing the sound, but he sees me; that much is true. He sprints toward me, sweeping me off my feet as if I was nothing more than a rag doll. "My God, this isn't real. Are you real?" he asks, his delight obvious through ragged breaths.

I cover my mouth, my hand trembling like a fish out of water because I'm not sure I can answer him without bursting into tears. I nod with a definitive yes and he pulls me in closer, feathering his nose against mine. "I can't believe you're in my arms." His words are soft, raspy, and deep—the sound makes my heart blip. Everett's lips onerously consume mine, and I forget how to breathe. I'm terrified that I am imagining this all.

The shouts, catcalls, and screeches surrounding us tell me this can't be happening in only my imagination. This isn't how life works. Dreams don't just come true in this way, but if they do, I'm not letting him go. I wrap my arms around his neck, squeezing so tightly I could be strangling him. He lowers me down and loops his arm behind me, holding me against his chest where I hear how hard his heart is beating. I can feel the pulse against my cheek.

"I just got your letters today," I tell him.

He stares down at me with disbelief. "I just got yours today too. We arrived here only a couple days ago. I didn't want to come to this thing tonight, but my guys—"

"The other girls dragged me here too," I tell him.

"Thank goodness," he says, kissing me again. "Oh, Lizzie, I am overwhelmed and in shock. I can't believe you're here. I'm here. We need to leave right now."

"You read my mind," I tell him.

"But first, you need to meet my guys, and I want to meet your friends. Then we'll tell them we're leaving and not to follow us," Everett says, sweeping his hand down the side of my face. I'm melting into the warmth of his arms, feeling alive again for the first time since I spoke to him last.

Everett takes my hand and pulls me toward the front of the crowd as he wraps his arms around my neck. "Fellas, this here, is my Lizzie. I didn't know she was here. This is unreal."

The men all look just as surprised as Everett. "This is your Lizzie?" One of them asks.

"This is my girl," Everett says.

"Romeo, here, has not shut up about you in a damn year. We kept thinking he'd run out of things to say about you, but no, they just kept coming. We were wondering if you even existed or if our man was just losing his mind."

One of the other guys slaps the outspoken one in the gut. "It's a pleasure to meet you, sweetheart. It's nice to see our Lieutenant looking a little less like a wet sock."

"Everett, a wet sock?" I question.

"He is one lovesick puppy, Miss," another says.

"All right. I think we are just about done here. I'm taking off. Will you fellas be okay finding your way back to camp?"

"Yes, Sir."

"Hot damn. I think the question is, will you ever find your way back to camp?" one of the boys asks.

"He's going to be walking on water tomorrow, gentleman."

Everett pulls me away from the comments, ones I'm enjoying entirely too much. "What a friendly group of gentlemen," I say, tugging Everett's arm.

"Yeah, they're—ah-real sweet talkers."

"Um, hello, *miss-I-don't-talk-to-men*. Are you going to introduce us to your famous Hollywood picture-person friend?" It shouldn't come as a shock when Beverly comes out of nowhere, stepping right in front of us so we can't move. She is the one person I don't want to see right now.

"Everett Anderson," he says, introducing himself to Beverly. Everett reaches his hand out to shake hers.

In true Beverly style, she takes Everett's hand and curtsies as if he's royalty. Then her hands move to her hair as her teeth pinch down against her bottom lip. "I can't tell a lie; I was sure Lizzie was giving us a story when telling us about you. We all kind of figured she's just a prude virgin, scared of—"

Everett clears his throat and wraps me into his arm a little tighter. "You know, I've heard so much about you, Beverly, none of which I assumed to be a story, of course, but Lizzie has gone on and on about you." Everett places a kiss on my cheek and clasps my hand between his.

Beverly fans her hand to the side of her face. "Has she now?" she asks. "Well, hopefully all good things." She bears a smile showing all her teeth, looking like a horse reaching for a carrot.

"Good things?" Everett repeats with a curt smirk. He gives me a quick glance, then looks back at Beverly. "Absolutely none. Now, if you'll excuse us." Everett pulls me toward the back of the room, and I feel like I'm walking on air as my hand melts into his.

"Have I told you how wonderful you are yet?" I ask him.

"Not as wonderful as the look we just left on that twit's face," Everett follows.

"Maggie and Isabel are right over there, waiting to be swept off their feet by a couple of soldiers. The two of them have no luck in the romance department, but they aren't giving up hope."

Everett follows me over to the girls and they both seem to choke on their drinks as they spot me.

"Holy moly," Maggie says. "You're here in real life." She reaches over and pokes Everett's arm.

Isabel steps forward and gives Everett a friendly hug. "Thank goodness you're here. Our girl has been worried sick about you. If anyone deserves a spark of happiness right now, it's Lizzie—the fiercest little spitfire we have in our unit."

Everett glances down at me with a cute grin. "I am not surprised to hear this, not in the slightest."

"Well, if you two don't mind, I think we're going to split. I'll see you later, okay?"

"Take your time, sweetie. Enjoy every moment with this gorgeous man. Gosh, I'm jealous," Isabel says.

Everett's hand tightens around mine, signaling his discomfort.

"Oh, don't do anything I wouldn't do," Maggie shouts out.

I look over my shoulder, finding Isabel clapping her hand over her mouth.

When the cool air from outside touches my face, the only words that come to mind are, "What do you say we run as far away as we can right now?"

"I'm not sure that would be far enough, but yes," he says.

41

MARCH 1944

TO FIND a night when the sky isn't falling with tears seems to be a miracle during the springtime here, but maybe the heavens above are offering Everett and me a break, like the eye of a storm, for a peaceful moment to reconnect. Our fingers are woven together, and our palms are inseparable as we stroll down the cobblestone streets. We're both quiet at first, as if we're strangers again, but I know this isn't the reason for our silence.

"I want to know everything, and I haven't had the time to read all of your letters since last spring. This feels like a dream, Everett."

Everett lifts my hand and places a warm kiss on my knuckles. "It may take me a lifetime to tell you everything, Lizzie, but what I can say is that the heaviness in my chest—the questions weighing me down with wonder if you were all right and safe—is more of a relief than I could ever ask for."

"I can certainly agree with that," I tell him. "It feels as though a thousand pounds have been lifted off my heart. I haven't had a worry-free moment since I left you in Oahu."

We find a bench along the side of some shops and Everett lifts my hand, allowing me to take a seat first.

"I've seen a lot," he begins. "It's mostly been during the last few months. I can't erase the scenes from my head, no matter how many times I try to convince myself they are fictional sets from a screenplay. The worst of it is at night, though, when things are quieter. The guys aren't talking and we're all just laying on our bunks in the dark. That's when the images burn through my mind as if they are happening all over again, right at that moment."

I take Everett's hand within mine and hold it against my chest.

"I'm not at will to discuss where we have been. It could be dangerous for both of us, but I've witnessed the depths of despair, the truth behind this war, and a direct view into Hitler's agenda. The fights are deadly, the attacks are overwhelming and never ending. Our enemies do not plan to give up this fight and my confidence is waning by the day."

I place one of my hands on Everett's chin and coerce him to look at me, but when his eyes meet mine, the glow from the street lantern shows an empty reflection—a stillness as he appears to stare through me. Something is missing or broken within his soul. "I haven't seen much here, aside from the casualties from a unit of airmen after an air raid. I feel like I'm waiting for the worst to come as the days crawl by in slow measures of long pauses."

"Doll, listen to me. I know that what I'm about to say, you will not take lightly because you are not the kind of woman who settles for an easy path, but the thought of you seeing what I have seen is what keeps me up at night long after the horrific images fade away. The place where I was is terrible. They're torturing Jewish people, killing them on the streets for no reason. These innocent souls are being deported to death camps and work camps. I've watched their tormented faces as they're captured and dragged away, often in front of their family. This war has taken an even more lethal turn, and it's clear that one of the primary objectives is to eliminate the Jewish race. I love you for who you are, but knowing you are a Jewish woman who could easily be standing in the same place of those I have seen tortured or killed, has brought me to the brink of harm's way more times than I can count. I have lunged at opportunities to intervene altercations between a Nazi soldier and a Jewish man or woman. But even though I may temporarily set a person free, reality always hits me after. It's hard to process the fact that I'm only helping a few people when millions are targeted."

I'm not ignorant to what has been happening in enemy

countries around Europe. The radio has enlightened me more than I wish most days, but what am I to do at this moment? It wasn't until last year that we found out Hitler's ultimate agenda is genocide. Fortunately, I've been moving back and forth between Scotland and England most of this time, but I'm aware how fast our unit can ship off into a different direction. "I'm American, and I don't have papers stating I'm Jewish," I tell Everett.

"Do not give your name to anyone who isn't with your unit. Lie if you need to."

I have always refused to buckle in the name of fear, and I pride myself on being stronger than others' thoughts and opinions, but what he is describing is only the tip of the iceberg to what's happening.

"I will lie if I'm—when it's necessary," I tell him.

"Beverly, is she a threat in any way?"

"Beverly," I repeat, swallowing the lump in my throat.

"I was afraid of that."

"I'm not sure she would do something to endanger me, but if there was a situation where it came down to her life or mine, she would spit out my last name without hesitation."

Everett stands up from the bench as if the seat burst into flames. "You must distance yourself from her, Elizabeth. I'm not sure how much longer your unit is going to remain in this area, and when you move, I am doubtful it will be a safe place."

"How can I do such a thing when we are in the same unit and billeted in the same house? Four of us have remained together since we left the United States. It would be impossible to avoid her."

Everett paces, his hands clasped behind his back. "Has she said much else to you after her blatant ridicule last year?"

I stand from the bench to stop him in his step. "She's made statements alluding to the subject but nothing so blunt as to her original comment when she told me I was endangering our entire unit." I place my hand on Everett's chest. "Stop."

He lowers his chin, offering a downward gaze. "I'm scared, Lizzie." Everett cups his hands around my cheeks ever so gently. "Despite the amount of times fear has consumed me with thoughts of something happening to you this past year, I convinced myself you were still okay, somehow. But finding you tonight, makes me wonder if it's fate; that we were meant to meet here at this exact moment so I could say what I need to say to you. Believe me when I tell you I don't want to cause you unnecessary fear, but if I keep my thoughts to myself, I could never forgive myself if anything were to happen. Whatever you must do to keep yourself safe, please, doll, you have to do it."

I reach up behind my neck and unclasp the necklace I have not gone a day without wearing since Mom passed away. The feeling of the gold chain parting from my skin feels like I'm pulling apart two magnets intended to stay as one unit. Everett closes his eyes while watching me remove the jewelry. I take his hand and turn it over to drop the necklace into his palm. "Keep this safe for me."

Everett closes his fist around my most treasured belonging and places his forehead down against mine. "Lizzie, I will care for this until we are back together and safe. I know the special meaning it has for you because it is a part of your mom."

I pull in a fluttering breath. "What now?"

Everett takes my hand and leads us across the street. "What time do you have to report for duty in the morning?"

"Zero five hundred hours," I respond, silently questioning where we are going.

"Okay," he says, looking around as if searching for watchful eyes. "They have billeted you to a house, you said?"

"Yes, it's located just outside of Glasgow."

"How far away is that from here?" Everett takes a second to glance down at his watch as if he's trying to figure out how to make the unthinkable work.

"The train took a little over an hour. Why, what are you planning?"

"We're in transit but recovering before our next destination, not far from here—just far enough. I don't know how long we'll stay put, but I can't waste a moment of this time, Lizzie. Take me home with you right now. I'll ride the train back in the morning." The thought of morning coming so soon makes my heart ache, but I'm the one who has always demanded that we live for the moment and nothing more.

"There is no way I can waste time sleeping tonight," I say.

"I wasn't planning to sleep much either," he replies, taking my hand and guiding us toward the train station.

* * *

The sheets that have done nothing more than gnarl and wrinkle against my nightly tosses and turns are pulling tightly, tangling around us. The fabric feels like a cool silk against my hot skin.

"I wonder when the others will be back?" Everett asks, sweeping his fingers through my loose strands of hair. "Will they mind if there's a man in the house?"

"Mind?" I question. "For every lewd sound I have overheard in this house, I can say, without a doubt, there are no rules about the guests we have."

"Guests you say?" Everett questions with a quirk to his brow.

I didn't mean to make him question whether I have brought a man here. "No, no, I have not had any company here if that's what you're wondering."

"I wasn't," he says. "It's just—I didn't think women were as hungry as the men I spend my days and nights with. We don't have many opportunities for rest, but they take full advantage of any free moments."

"They?" I question in retaliation.

"Yes, doll-face. Only 'they.'"

"Well, it isn't all four of the girls. It's mostly Beverly and on occasion, Isabel, if she finds a friendly Brit."

Everett doesn't seem as if he's paying attention to my words anymore as he strokes the back of his finger down the side of my cheek. He's gaze falls to my lips.

"Someday, I want to spend every night of my life with you, like this," he murmurs, sending shivers up my spine.

This is exactly how I imagine a life with him; late night talks and whispers of sweet nothings while lying in the moon's glowing embrace.

"We will have a lifetime," I tell him, trying to convince myself of an ending to a love story that the author hasn't finished writing yet. "Like this: intertwined, warm, and protected by the walls that surround us."

"I couldn't imagine anything more perfect," he says, leaning in to claim my lips again.

* * *

I tried my hardest to stay awake all night, fighting every yawn and long blink, but it isn't until the morning light peeks through the window, and feeling Everett's lips against my forehead that I know I wasted precious hours.

"I love you, doll. I will be back as soon as I can for as long as I have here."

"Everett," I utter. "I love you so much." My voice is hoarse, and my head is still in a haze. "These last ten hours have been like a dream, and more than I could have asked for, but I will take whatever more time you can offer no matter when that might mean."

With one last kiss, the air current from his movement brings a chill to my body and the sound of the creaking door stings the inside of my ears. My chest feels deflated and my pulse quickens. Once again, I am empty inside, wishing I could hold on to a feeling of comfort, something I only have when we are together.

42

JUNE 1944

THE EARLY SUMMER season in Glasgow is the most pleasant time of the year. The wavering scent of flowers and greenery fill the air, and there are more days of blue skies than not. It's pleasant not to feel the deep chill within my bones when I leave for the hospital each morning. We all have different assignments today and various times to report to duty, but I won't mind the quiet on the train ride this morning.

My evening rendezvous with Everett ended during the latter part of April when he moved further south. We are about six hours away from each other now, but over the weeks that followed his relocation, we were able to meet a few times in the middle for a late dinner. The last time we saw each other was in the middle of May, but the ability to remain in contact with him has been enough of a relief that I can live with the distance and brief encounters.

The walk to the train station isn't more than a few blocks down the road, but I wasn't expecting a delay to hold me up from the train I need to catch. A car skids to a stop beside me.

"Doll-face, get in, right away."

A gasp catches in my throat when I see Everett in the driver's seat. "Everett, what in the world are you doing here?"

"I'll explain. Get in. I'll take you to the hospital."

This certainly isn't like our typical long-awaited hellos, which means something is happening or has happened. There's urgency in his voice and a lack of excitement in his eyes. My stomach gnarls with wonder as I slip into the passenger seat of a car that smells of stale pipe tobacco. There are cigarette ashes scattered along the dashboard in a thick layer of dust. Questioning who the car belongs to is the least of my concerns, but Everett hasn't had a mode of transportation aside from the train, like me.

"Have you been driving all night?" I question, closing the door.

"Yes, I've been on the road since the very early morning. Baby, I'm leaving the United Kingdom. There's a mission I have to lead, and the situation is volatile and ever-changing, along with some unpredictable orders from up the ranks."

Everett is driving, his words are forming, but I can't see the look in his eyes. It's the only way I can determine the level of trouble he's facing. I assume he's avoiding eye contact for that reason. "Today?"

"Yes, as soon as I drop you off. I must get back to England by noon. We're leaving this afternoon."

"Where are you going, Everett? Can you tell me, please?"

When Everett is nervous, he checks the rear-view mirror more frequently as if someone might be following us, but it's never the case. I believe it's his way of avoidance.

"Have you heard anything about your brothers' whereabouts?"

Everett is changing the subject. He isn't planning to tell me where he's going, which is the typical since he's sworn to secrecy for protection, but it's just us here in the car. There are no letters going through the mail or tapped connections during a phone call.

"No, Dad said they were safe. That's all I know. Everett, please tell me what's going on."

"You're going to be moving soon as well. You aren't to know any of this, Elizabeth. Orders have not come down the ranks yet."

"What? Where will I be going?"

"We're both being moved to France," he says.

With the dream I have always had to travel, this feels like a torturous tease. As a child, I dreamed of visiting the Eiffel Tower,

Versailles, the Louvre, but France is not just Paris and I'm sure wherever I'm going won't be a part of the country I want to be in. Germany invaded France over four years ago and still occupies the country.

"We're going to be pushing the Germans out, aren't we?" I ask.

"The military is going to need the support of medical care."

Everett answers each question with indirect answers, which just stokes the flames of fear running through my mind.

"You're going to be in danger." I'm not asking; I'm stating the obvious.

"I have confidence in what we are doing and the team I will work with are trained for the situation we're facing. You shouldn't worry about us, but I need you to prepare for a vast change in scenery from what you've become accustomed to. Do you recall our conversation about lying about your last name?"

"Yes," I answer, squeezing my hands together as I watch the blood pool in my fingertips.

"All you have to do is keep your head down and do what's necessary. There will not be any more USO events. The country is in grave danger and locked down. The rules and restrictions are strict and unyielding, and you mustn't go outside of the encampment. Promise me, you will stay within US military confines? I know your wild sense of curiosity gets the best of you sometimes, and I would never ask this of you unless it was a matter of life or death, but it is and I need you to follow orders, please, Lizzie."

Everett must think I have taken liberties over the last two years to fulfill my need for adventure, but truthfully, I have not wandered off anywhere, no matter where I have been. This isn't the same as looking for a hidden beach in Hawaii or a gem of a view only the locals know about. I'm smart enough to not go looking for trouble in a foreign place.

"Of course, I will follow orders, Everett. You can't think I would be so reckless and foolish as to act like a tourist in a war-torn country being overrun by the enemy?"

Everett glances over at me for a brief second, and I see the look of anguish in his eyes.

"I know we see life differently sometimes, so I needed to say this for the sake of my sanity."

"Everett, I will be fine," I reply with a sharp edge to my words.

I don't want to feel angered at Everett's questions or assumptions that I'm not taking the situation for what it is. We're in the middle of a war, but he must still see me as that free-willed girl, who doesn't take orders from anyone, running down the beach in Hawaii. "Okay," he replies.

Silence and heavy breaths take over the rest of our ride. This can't be the way we leave things. I know his comments and requests came from his heart, but I need to know his safety should be his top concern at the moment. He will be in more danger than me.

"Please do not worry about me, Everett. I need to know that you are going to focus on whatever you are dealing with."

"Of course," he says. His words fall short, almost in an authoritative tone.

Everett pulls up in front of the hospital and I'm supposed to step out of the car like this is common and not out of the ordinary for us.

"Okay then, maybe I'll see you in France," I say, my words cold and tart.

"Lizzie," he says, grabbing my hand before I open the door. "I'm sorry. Look, this isn't good. For either of us, okay? This war is about to take a turn for the worse. I can't lie. I don't know what either of us will face in the coming weeks."

My eyes threaten to fill with tears, but I inhale and stare up to the metal ceiling of the car.

"Okay. I understand."

"Take this envelope and keep it safe—keep it in your journal. The unit I'm leaving with written down inside, and a few other things I hope you will not need. Your necklace is also inside. I need you to keep that in a hidden pocket of a uniform you aren't wearing during your time in France. It's not safe with me at the moment. I can't explain this in much more detail, but please do not keep it on you."

This time, the tears come without warning and it's one of the few times I have cried in front of Everett. I'm not one to use emotions to express myself. I find words to be more practical but I'm experiencing more than pain, more than fear, more than despair, and there are no adequate words to describe how I feel. Everett pulls me across the seat and under his arm, nuzzling my head against his chest.

"We've made it this far, Lizzie. Let's not throw in the towel. We can get through this too."

For the first time in the last two years, I don't feel confident in what I can handle. Until now, I don't believe I've even seen a fraction of what Everett has. I feel weak, and it's maddening because I need to be strong.

"I love you," I whisper.

"Always, doll-face. Don't forget how powerful those clouds are, okay? If you need me, you know I'm there."

My body shudders and I sniffle as I tilt my head back to kiss him. He reaches for my cheek, but with a sense of reluctance. I feel his body stiffen beneath his touch as he brushes his lips against mine. It isn't a passionate goodbye like we've shared so many times before. This is just a goodbye.

43

JULY 1944

WE CAN DESCRIBE the front lines as a meeting point between two sides; us and the enemy, and that is where our evacuation hospital now is, so we can take in the vast number of casualties that we anticipate. We're five miles from Beachhead in Normandy. Walls no longer surround us while we tend to patients. Instead, we have set up a camp full of hand-secured canvas tents where we will sleep, eat, and treat. Large sets of artillery surrounding the camp are in place to protect us, but with the German planes cruising through the skies every night, each minute I'm alive feels like a blessing.

All the military units in the vicinity are in a constant battle, and our nursing personnel works into two shifts. All of us have an assignment to various tents to keep casualties organized and handled with standard routine. I'm tending to the shock unit which is at capacity each day. Many tests are necessary to diagnose and treat the varying degrees of shock, since the source of a patient's condition is not always obvious.

There isn't a moment to stop and blink, which is best for my current state of mind, and my downtime should be for sleeping, but I'm not sure many of us can close our eyes without seeing the horrific visions from our days.

Several weeks have passed since the passive goodbye Everett and I shared in front of the hospital in Scotland. I know he was deploying to France, but I know nothing more. Whatever isn't occurring in front of us isn't news we often come across. Communication is sparse and when we have a few seconds to take a breath and think, we can only manage to wonder how much worse things will get. And when I see our planes whizzing through the sky, all I can do is watch and wonder if one of them is Everett, but I will never know.

My tent is unusually quiet with most of my patients being unconscious or drowsy from head trauma or other injuries. I'm constantly monitoring bodily temperatures, infusing the intravenous bags with pain medication, and ensuring I keep the men warm and comfortable. When I see a man with a lifeless stare, I wonder if they are on the brink of death, silently whispering their goodbyes to their loved ones.

"We need to stop those bastards. Do you hear me?" Herbert Donning cries out. He's a member of the infantry who pushed forward through Beachhead against the Germans. They shot him multiple times and beat him close to death before anyone could rescue him. His serious wounds are on the mend, but psychologically, he seems lost in a faraway place we are having trouble pulling him back from.

I place the back of my hand on his forehead, finding his temperature to be holding steady in a normal range, but he's inconsolable. "Herbert, sweetheart, look at me," I tell him, taking a seat on the edge of his cot. "No one is going to hurt you here. You're safe and everything is going to be okay."

"They shot him right in the face like he was nothing more than a tin can. But, no, they had not inflicted enough damage, so they had to keep going. They mutilated him and didn't stop until they determined he was dead. But they will not stop. No. Until we're all like that—with no faces." Herbert doesn't blink while he speaks. "I tried to help, Miss. I swear I did, but they took the others."

"Herbert, what does that mean?" I ask, trying to understand so I can figure out how to calm him down.

"They're prisoners. Our men. They took them. They're going to torture and kill them."

We haven't heard news about any of our men becoming

prisoners, but that doesn't mean it hasn't happened. Herbert hasn't been making sense with everything he says, and it's hard to decipher what might be fact or something conjured up in his mind.

"Someone will find them," I say.

"Without the airborne. We need our pilots."

His words shoot through me like a dagger, but I have to take a deep breath and remind myself how many airborne units we have, as well as pilots, and paratroopers. "You're right, Herbert, we do."

"We'll never get home."

Herbert continues talking in circles until he falls into a trance-like stare, as he does every few hours.

I'm warming bottles for newer patients who I haven't regulated temperatures for yet when Beverly storms into my tent. "Did you hear?"

I shrug at her dramatization. "Hear what, Beverly?"

"There's news that some of the four-hundred bodies no one can find are being kept as prisoners somewhere. I overheard a commander mention two units have missing men. It was 105th or 505th, or maybe 501st regiment. Shoot."

I can't tell if she's being sincere or trying to trip me up. It seems to be her latest motivation since our captain promoted me to first Lieutenant, and she has not received a higher rank yet.

"When you have more facts, let me know," I tell her.

"What if it's Everett's regiment? What if Everett is missing or worse?" Beverly continues. "He's part of one of those airborne units, isn't he?"

"I need to focus on what I'm doing right now. Like I said, when you have more information, please let me know," I repeat, trying to maintain my composure until she walks away from me. "Poor Everett," she mutters before leaving the tent.

I feel like a hammer is beating against the outside of my chest as I try to hold myself up and push her words out of my head. Everett is a pilot which means he wasn't jumping from planes.

They could have shot him down, though.

44

SEPTEMBER 1944

IT WAS TRUE. It was the one time Beverly had accurate information. At the time of her whispers, I didn't know how many US soldiers had become prisoners of war. I wasn't aware of the direction my life was about to take. Because I am not Everett's wife or kin, I am not entitled to the details of his whereabouts — if he even has a location. I'm unsure if Everett is dead or a prisoner, but I have received confirmation that he is missing. Through personal investigational tactics, I have questioned patients who are part of Everett's unit, and they confirmed his plane was shot down over water. No one knows if he jumped or — I can't fathom the alternate.

It's been six weeks since learning this information.

I'm a shell of a person, using the parts of my brain required to keep the men under my care alive, but during the hours I should be asleep, I weep against a rolled up sleeping bag until there are no more tears.

Some days I ponder if I'm even alive while walking back and forth between tents scattered across dead grass, areas painted with our blood again and again. I consider this life to be a form of hell, one I didn't know existed. I've broken all rules and sent letters home to inform Dad of the situation, using as few words as possible. He hasn't written back, which tells me he wants me to stop writing. I'm aware of the problems compromised communication can cause, but I've become a selfish person over the last couple months—a mean, spiteful, human being trapped in the body of a caring nurse.

I watch men in shock, wishing I could trade places with them, even with their severe injuries and amputations, knowing they may never regain full cognition or mobility again. I cannot compare their pain to mine, but to imagine anything worse than this guttural ache that never goes away is incomprehensible.

The weight on my chest makes me feel like my body might cave in, every minute of every day. I'm not sure how much longer I can go on like this, like a mouse in a maze, looking for a way out, but unable to escape. It could go on like this for years.

When I reach moments of utter exhaustion and pain in the pit of my stomach from vomiting up everything I swallow, I excuse myself from the medical tent, walk over to the nestled trees and fall to my knees.

It's not a habit I want to continue, but one I can't prevent. I've had to remind myself I'm only human, and I have been witnessing the most horrific atrocities day after day for months. I want to become numb to it all, but the agony is relentless. And worse, I regret every decision I have ever made regarding this pursuit of purpose. It's clear to me now that the consequence is a lifetime sentence.

"I thought I saw you run into the woods. What on earth are you doing out here, Lizzie?" Nancy—who is my only saving grace among this tragedy, is always where I need her, right when I am at my lowest moment of despair. She is like an angel, and sometimes I wonder if she truly exists or if she is a figment of my confounded imagination. "You know better than to come in here alone. Those Nazis are lurking in every dark shadow."

A dry heave rivets up my esophagus and I wrap my arms around the tree in front of me for support.

"Shh, okay, okay," Nancy says, rubbing her hand in circles around my back. "There is nothing left for you to get rid of, sweetie. You aren't eating enough to survive at this point." Nancy lifts me to my feet and walks us out of the woods, back into the compound of canvas tents. Her embrace is holding me up as I lean my cheek against her chest, wanting to cry to fill the concave feeling in my chest with pain rather than the hollow air. "Way back when we first arrived in Scotland, you told me about this trick you had with staring into the clouds to find what you were looking for."

I remember the conversation. I was trying to help her when she was having a touch of trouble settling into our unforgiving lifestyle. It was before I knew her daughter had passed away a few years prior, but she described a type of pain I was familiar with—a longing to be somewhere—a place I can't describe.

I spent years trying to define a feeling of loss. The only comparison I found was to a flower losing its roots—the source of life. The detachment would lead to wilting petals falling to the ground—a place to wait, shrivel up, and eventually decompose. If a flower severs from its roots, it cannot live. When Mom died, I was the severed flower torn from its roots. Yet, I needed to carry on and continue to grow into a respectable young woman.

The unfairness between humanity and nature made me angry, so I longed for a better understanding of life, and did so by spending days upon days staring up at the clouds. I watched them form into responses to my questions. I came to depend on the clouds to give me a sign. Then Everett caught me in the act one day, and he found the same sense of contentment from within the cloud's messages.

"Of course, I remember," I reply.

"Look up into the sky, Lizzie. What do you see?"

I can't see anything. I've tried so many times when there wasn't a sky full of clouds, but the white puffs of moisture floating through the sky resemble nothing anymore. I can't find the answers or signs anywhere in the sky. "There's nothing—just a void."

"Well, I see something," she says, pointing up above our heads.

I stare at the cluster of clouds, but it looks like nothing more than a paint splotch.

"That's a flying elephant, if you ask me," she says.

My shoulders drop and I take a step back to look her in the eyes. "What did you say you saw?"

"Well, look for yourself. It looks like a flying elephant." I swallow hard and peer back up at the white puffs, finding a long trunk and floppy ears like Dumbo. The film came out the year I met Everett, and I figured that was the reason he told me that's what he saw in the sky, but I couldn't see anything that looked like a flying elephant that day. I thought he was playing along with my silly game of finding objects in the sky.

"I see it," I tell her.

"Well, I can't tell you what a flying elephant means, but it isn't the void you are speaking about."

"It means something to me," I whisper.

"The moment you think you can't take anything more; life has a way of pushing you a little harder before everything falls into place. Trust me. It doesn't always make sense at the time, but it will someday."

"Do you think he's dead?"

Nancy places her hands on my shoulders and squeezes. "Lizzie, when your mom died, what did you feel inside?"

The thought of recalling those moments will not help my current state of mind. "It was as if I had been holding hundreds of balloons and then released them. They almost pulled me with it, but I let them go and watched them fly away until they weren't visible anymore. It was like I knew she was still there, but I just couldn't see her. It might not make sense, but it's the only way I can describe the feeling."

"I know exactly what you mean, but look at me, sweetie, I know for a fact that you are still holding onto those balloons for Everett, which means in your heart, you know he's still alive. Lizzie, I don't know much, but I know my gut is more honest with me than any word I've ever heard," she says.

Part of me wishes she wouldn't offer me false hope. The other part wants to take what she is saying and hold on to it with dear life. "It seems impossible to assume he's okay. It's been almost three months."

"Don't give up yet," she says.

Nancy places a kiss on my temple and walks back toward her assigned tent.

I take in the deepest breath I can and return to my patients for the remaining two hours until my shift is over.

* * *

It's hard to walk out of the tent before dusk, knowing I'm leaving these men in their battered condition. It feels as though I'm abandoning them sometimes, even though someone else is taking my place, but I leave them all with a smile and a promise to return tomorrow, hoping it's enough to keep them going through the night.

The walk between my medical tent and the tent we sleep beneath is just across the field from each other. The path is just long enough to take in a few breaths of fresh air and to convince myself I'm hungry enough for whatever food they're offering tonight.

A convoy of US vehicles skids over the dirt lot, forcing anyone in its path to freeze with wonder. "American POWs—we need hands," one of the soldier's shouts from his open window.

Men are running from every direction to help the five vehicles I'm facing. I'm frozen, unable to breathe, blink, or think straight. Someone is walking toward me; the shadow of a man is all I can make out. I turn to look behind me, wondering if there is someone else this person is looking for, but they are heading in my direction.

With the sun falling behind the horizon, there is a sharp glare and until the man is directly in front of me, I didn't know I was staring at Lewis. I cup my hands over my mouth and fall into his arms. "What—you're here—how—"

"Shh, shh. Come on. Come with me." Lewis helps me over to the nearest tent where there are rows of cots lined up for the troops.

"You're here," I say again.

"I've been here, kiddo, just offshore. Are you in one piece?" Lewis kneels and pushes me away from him like he did when I was much smaller than him as a child. "You're not hurt, are you?"

"No, not physically," I mutter. "Lewis, I thought I was stronger. I thought I could do this, but I want to go home."

"Everyone feels that way during combat," he says.

"I think Everett is—"

"He's not. We have him."

"What?" I squeak with the remainder of sound I have left in my voice.

"He's not in good shape, Lizzie, but I think we got him in time."

I turn, ready to run for him, with no idea where to look, but I need to be where he is. "Take me to him. Lewis, take me there, please."

"Lizzie, stop."

"What? Why?" I shout.

"Everett was a prisoner, and he was tortured. He doesn't look the way he did when you saw him last. I need to prepare you for what you're about to face, and this is by far the last thing I would ever want you to have to witness. You must understand."

"I don't care what he looks like, Lewis. I just want to be with him."

"That's the unstoppable girl I know," he says, pinching my cheek. "He needs you."

45

SEPTEMBER 1944

OVER THE PAST TWO YEARS, I thought I had seen it all, or at least, the worst of it. After being witness to the most horrific of injuries, I thought nothing could ever suck the air from my lungs again, but to approach someone I love and face the unimaginable requires a type of bravery I'm not sure I have. As I walk beside Lewis, I try to maintain my composure, but it's a facade. My heart pounds like a drum as I step closer and closer to what could be the end of my world. "Is he conscious?"

"He's—well, yes, somewhat. However, you should try to prepare yourself. He isn't making much sense when he tries to speak," Lewis explains, keeping his voice soft. He's being as gentle as he can with me, knowing full well that I'm no different at this moment than a grenade after I have pulled the safety ring.

"What are his injuries?" I continue, ignoring his attempt to walk on eggshells.

"We aren't sure of his condition or prognosis yet. The immediate priority was to get him here to the hospital as quickly as we could. We can see the external injuries, but what's happening internally is yet to be diagnosed."

"Can you at least tell me what you know? Please don't speak in riddles, Lewis."

"All right. I'll give it to you straight. He has multiple contusions, a broken ankle, and several injured ribs. There could be head trauma, but to what extent, is not yet clear. What is obvious is that he has been starving and dehydrated beyond what most men would survive. The long-term effects of his injuries — well, we just don't know." Lewis's explanation is uncoated and sharp, but there is no way to lighten the description that I asked for. If I wasn't already aware that I have nothing left in my stomach to vomit up, I would prepare to become sick.

"I missed you," I tell Lewis.

"Me too, kid. It's been a long time, but your letters have made me laugh more times than I can count. I know it looks like we're losing this war, but we aren't. We're doing good things, better than what you can see."

"Yeah, you've said that in your letters," I say, elbowing him gently in the side. "I'm having trouble seeing much past the deaths and injuries, though."

Lewis takes my chin in his hand. "You are Mom, and you can do this. You hear me, Elizabeth?" I try to swallow against my dry throat, but I feel like choking. I nod in response. "I wish I could stay with you, but I'm not supposed to be here. I just — I need to help and make sure you are okay. James and I fought over who would go. I won this time." Out of habit, I roll my eyes, finding out that he and James are somehow together and still fighting over everything.

"I should have figured as much."

We're approaching one of the intensive care tents where we tend to the most serious injuries to first. I'm lightheaded as we step into the cloaked, humid space filled with body lined cots. I would do anything for more air than I can currently take in, but I'm not sure I'll ever be able to take a full breath again until I know Everett is going to be okay.

"He's lost a lot of weight," Lewis says.

Everett was always lean, but with a muscular physique. He was the picture of good health.

Lewis places his hand on my back to turn me toward Everett's cot. My heart stops beating for a moment as I approach his side. He's pale, but scabbed with what looks like burn marks, his lips are bluish, but cracked and dry. The sunken dip in his cheeks and temples is intense, and though a sheet is covering most of his chest, his collarbone is far more defined than someone who has been starving for just a few weeks. It looks like he hasn't eaten in months.

But he's still beautiful.

"Hey brother, look who I found," Lewis calls out to Everett.

Brother. That one simple word makes me weaker than I already am.

Everett struggles to open his eyelids, and his lips part slightly.

"Baby," I call out. "It's Lizzie. I'm here." I fall to my knees and carefully rest my cheek on his arm, not recognizing the scent or texture of his skin. His hands are much larger than mine and when we would intertwine our fingers, his hand would cover mine as if he had a bear claw in comparison. Now, our fingers look similar in width, but Everett's are still much longer.

"Liz—" he mumbles.

I lift my head and place the back of my hand on the side of his. "Everett, I'm here, and I'm not going anywhere."

"It's—bye. I need—I—"

"No goodbyes. Don't say that to me. You need to rest. You're safe." This is what I say to all the men when they arrive in my care, knowing my words aren't always the truth. There's no way to provide an honest statement about anyone's safety in the conditions we're in. None of us can call ourselves safe. We could be the target of an air raid, dropped on us at any moment if one bypasses our artillery.

"How many bags of intravenous fluid have you gotten into him?" I ask the attending nurse.

"This is the second bag," she says, checking the bag to see what's left.

I run my fingers through his hair, caked with dirt. He could never tolerate being dirty. Everett showered twice a day, most of the time. He never had an untrimmed nail or a hint of dirt on his hands. It must have been habits left over from the lifestyle he lived in Hollywood.

"Commander Laurel, do you mind if I sit with him for a while?" I ask, teetering on the edge of begging. "I'm off duty at the moment." I haven't spent much time with this commander. She came from a different unit when we moved to this location, but she has been in the Army a while and has earned respect with merit of her skills.

"Of course. He should be stable for the moment."

Lewis finds a folding chair and places it down next to Everett's side. "I'm going to go check in a few other tents," he says, placing a kiss on the top of my head. "I'll be back before I take off."

I grab Lewis's arm before he walks away. "Thank you," I say.

"You don't have to thank me, Elizabeth."

The commanding nurse and Lewis have left the vicinity, leaving me alone with Everett, a time in which I would normally fill his ears with as many stories as I could come up with. I don't want to stress him out though, so I trace my fingertips down the length of his arm.

"I saw a flying elephant in the sky earlier today. It was the first sign I saw that made me believe you were okay. I didn't want to give up hope, but I didn't know if I was trying to convince myself of something that might not be true."

Everett's eyelids flutter again, so I stand to make it easier for him to see me. "Tell me how you feel, sweetheart."

His blinks are slow and sluggish as he struggles to pull in a breath. "It hurts."

"What does? Your leg, ribs, or something else?"

"It hurts," he says again. "In my head."

Lewis said they weren't sure about head trauma yet, but I'm not sure if Everett is speaking about mental or physical pain.

"The memories?" I ask.

"No."

I slide my fingertips around his head, searching for bumps or wounds, but I don't feel any abnormalities. But that doesn't mean anything seeing as he was a prisoner for at least a couple months. I must think if he survived all this time, he would make it through this too, but that type of wishful thinking involves nothing more than hope.

I retrieve a clean cloth from the short stack on the rolling cart set off to the side and take a silver bowl to fill with some water. He's so parched and I can only imagine how uncomfortable he must be. I dip the cloth into the water and dab the fabric along his lips.

"Lizzie," he mumbles.

"I'm here," I say again.

"Lizzie."

If I could convince myself that he will improve and walk out of here someday, I would take comfort in that belief, but I've seen too many similar injuries end the other way. I want him to be the exception. I need him to be, but is it selfish to plead for such a thing at his expense? Maybe he wants to say goodbye so it will be over, and he can go home.

* * *

Two weeks have come and gone. We're still here in the critical ward tent. Everett has gained a small amount of weight back, and his coloring has returned to a fair pale, but his cognitive state has changed little. He will mutter a few different combinations of words and my name here and there, so I know he's still in there, but the medics and other nurses don't have high hopes for a dramatic change since so much time has passed. His level of shock is likely due to the internal damage we have yet to find. We are all trying to remain optimistic but with so little improvement, it's difficult to stay upbeat. I've spent every free minute during my off hours by his side, sometimes sleeping on the chair with my head resting on his arm. He knows I'm here, but I think he's locked inside of his head without the keys to get out.

* * *

"Just one more bite, sweetie." I spoon feed Everett the pureed fruits we've started giving in effort to take him off the intravenous fluid. It's great he's able to swallow the food on his own. We think it's an improvement, but his words are still few and far between, though they seem to make a bit of sense at times. It's been weeks and his bones have almost healed entirely. We should be seeing more progress than he is showing, but if there is one thing I have learned in my years of nursing school, it's that patience is sometimes the only cure.

"Doll," he mutters, turning his head to the side.

I place my hand in his. "Did you just call me doll?" He hasn't referred to me by any other name than Lizzie and it's never been in a way to call for my attention, more like just a word he mumbles.

"Doll," he says again.

"I love you," I say, smiling at his curious eyes.

He doesn't recognize me, or at least it doesn't feel like he does. The way he looks at me sometimes, I feel like nothing more than a stranger.

"Hi," he utters breathlessly.

"Hi," I reply. He seems proud of himself for carrying on this minor victory of a conversation. I'm proud of him too.

"How are you feeling?"

His eyes blink in a slow succession before closing. He takes several long naps a day—a stupor we can't seem to keep him from falling in and out of. Despite the progress, his diagnosis seems to change a bit each day. However, some days are worse than others, but the days that are better fill me with hope—hope that I need to hang on to.

* * *

The medics moved Everett into my tent; the shock unit where others like him are lying weak and unmoving in their cots. I spend my entire day under this canvas tarp, resisting sleep until my eyes lose the battle and close.

It's been a comfort being able to monitor him all day rather than just the hours I'm not working. However, seeing his stationary state for hours on end highlights a truth I'm still not willing to accept. He's shown improvement, despite how slowly it's happening. I have faith one of these days he will sit up on his own and ask me for a hot dog or a grinder. I wish and imagine it happening like I once dreamed of a day at the beach. It's all I want—the part of him that made him who he was to return.

"Doll-face," he calls out, his voice hoarse like always. "A cigarette."

I giggle at his statement. "What are you talking about, silly? You said smoking would cause you wrinkles at an early age. Do you remember that? You told me what it had done to your father."

"I don't have a father," he says.

"It was my mother." I'm not about to remind him that his mother is dead if it's slipped his mind, but he's confused about what he's saying.

"How about some water?"

"That's n—not nice," he says with a slight stutter.

"Nurses can't always be nice, especially when the patient is a little stubborn sometimes."

"I'm not stubborn. I'm famous."

That you are, Everett. I'm just not sure he recalls the timeline of when this was true.

"And charming," I whisper, pinching his chin.

"I love you. Marry me, doll."

I try to smile and convince myself he knows who I am, and that he knows he was in love with me before he became a prisoner. All I want to do is believe he knows what a marriage means and the meaning of having a life with someone, but I can't convince myself of this after everything we've been through. I don't know what part of his mind is intact and what part is not, but I pray he knows the person I am, the person I've been—the people we were together and the reason he's spouting off crazy words while lying in a cot under a medical tent.

46

NOVEMBER 1944

I'M GOING to try and spend more time in my cot for the sake of catching up on lost sleep. I won't be any good to Everett if I get sick, so a few hours of deep sleep, rather than quick naps in a chair by his bedside, are necessary. The fatigue has been affecting my ability to think on my toes and it's not fair to endanger any of my other patients either. As if there are bells ringing throughout the tent, I sit up straight like a jackknife at twenty minutes before zero five hundred hours, ready to take on my shift.

"I'm glad you slept in your bed last night," Isabel says, stretching her arms over her head. "You needed the rest. It's been almost six weeks of twenty-four-hour care for Everett. You're going to fall ill if you don't take better care of yourself."

"I did sleep well last night. I suppose it was a much-needed break after sleeping on those hard chairs in the shock unit. But comfort shouldn't matter when it comes to caring for the man I love, right?"

"He's doing better, Lizzie," Maggie speaks up.

"He is," I agree. "I'm just worried about the day he stops improving."

"You can't think like that," Isabel follows.

"Say, did you girls hear part of our unit is getting split up sometime this week?" Beverly grumbles with her mouth pressed into the side of her pillow.

"Where do you always hear these rumors?" Isabel asks her.

"Oh, you know. It pays to have an in with an officer," she sighs.

"I think she meant to say: it pays to have an officer in—" Isabel continues.

"Girls," Maggie interrupts, stopping the chatter before it goes any further. We all share a giggle which is refreshing since it doesn't happen often anymore.

We've done our best to keep our morale up, but between my silence, Maggie's nerves, and Beverly's obnoxious behavior, we've all been moody recently.

"I'll let you girls know if I hear anything more about a move," Beverly says. "Let's just hope Germany isn't next on our locations to go sightseeing. We don't want our precious Lizzie to be in that type of grave danger." A snort of laughter follows Beverly's unnecessary comments. There is nothing funny about what she's saying. We all know they could move us to Germany any time. We're pushing the lines forward and it will not end until we've accomplished what seems like the impossible.

Maggie, Isabel, and I roll our sleeping bags over our cots and tend to our hair before dressing and preparing to make our way to our assigned locations. Beverly strolls around late wherever she is going and somehow keeps herself out of trouble with the commanders and captains. It's annoying, because no one should receive special treatment when we are all struggling to get by each day.

"I hope you girls have a good day. Fingers crossed for no serious injuries and maybe some extra smiles on these boys' faces."

"Hear, hear," Isabel says, holding her tube of lipstick up in the air.

The weather is becoming colder by the day as we enter the autumn season and I'm dreading winter in these measly tents that do little to keep the chill out. I suppose something must change soon, anyway. It's not feasible to keep the patients in these conditions.

I've also heard mentions of Germany and the setup of another evacuation hospital, but it's all hearsay at this point. In any case, we'll be moving along with our patients and it's the only peace of mind I have at the moment.

I reach the shock unit tent and place my bag down on the hook just on the inside flimsy wall. "There she is," Everett drawls with a giddy, but weak smile.

"You're awfully alert this morning," I respond.

"He's been mumbling about you in his sleep all night," Alan, another shock patient follows. Alan is likely being released today or tomorrow. His injuries were minor, and the shock was because of a slight concussion he suffered upon falling.

"Is that right?" I question.

"My body is aching. I'm an old geezer, and I think I need a nurse." It's hard not to react to his words, so I lift a brow in Everett's direction. I'm beyond thrilled to hear his communication skills are improving so much, but we haven't been able to get him up and moving around yet and it's concerning after sustaining broken bones. The longer he's in bed, the weaker he'll become, not to mention the threat of blood clots and infection.

"How are you feeling this morning, Alan?"

"I'm well, thank you, Miss. I'm just hungry."

"Breakfast should be here shortly," I tell him.

I make my rounds, checking on the others, many of whom are still asleep or quietly staring at the ceiling. It's hard not to wonder what they're thinking about, but I presume it's either a replay of the horror they've endured or the dream of going back home to be with their families. As usual, I check body temperatures and fluff the pillows of those who are awake and not propped up. I'm also lucky enough to receive a few morning greetings. Watching these men make progress gets me through the days here.

I make my last stop at Everett's cot. "How are you feeling, sweetheart?" I run my fingers through his hair and then down the side of his face.

"How come he gets all that attention and all we get is a fluffed pillow?" Alan asks.

"She loves him more than you, bozo," Teddy, one of others speaks up. Teddy is close to moving out of the unit as well.

"Hush over there," I tell them.

"I want to get up," Everett says.

"We'll try again today," I say with a hopeful smile.

Everett places his hand on my arm and tugs weakly. "Come here," he says. I lean down, coming in close to the face I would love nothing more than to kiss until we are both left breathless. "I might go home. A doc said something."

"Home?" We haven't been able to transport anyone out of here because of the conditions, which is why we have been doing everything possible to be a functioning hospital at this camp site.

"I don't know," he says. "Somewhere."

"Maybe you misheard him."

Everett's face falls into a grimace. "Lizzie."

"Look at me," I say, grabbing his chin. "You have nothing to worry about."

"No one says I'll be okay," he mutters.

"I said you'll be okay, and you will be. Do you hear me?"

Everett attempts to stretch, seeming more uncomfortable than usual, so I help him readjust his position, spotting an angry red patch on his back. It's an ulcer with exposed tissue. I've been keeping him clean and moving him as often as possible but all of them go from hot-to-cold overnight. They're bundled up and then they often break into night sweats. The bedsores are almost unavoidable with some of them.

"I need to get you cleaned up. It looks like you have a bedsore," I tell Everett.

After compiling the items to disinfect the area, I come to find several more spots on his back. His temperature is higher than normal, and his blood pressure isn't where I'd like it to be. "I'm going to see about starting you on penicillin when the medic returns."

"I'm okay," Everett says through a groan as I clean the infected area with a cloth drenched in alcohol.

"This requires proper treatment. It's imperative, Everett." I'm concerned this might be the start of sepsis, and I am aware of the prognosis of a patient with a blood infection even under the best of circumstances which we don't have here. Just as things begin to improve, something else must go wrong.

"You're just worried," he says.

"I'm going to find the medic. I'll be right back."

The moment I step out of the tent, I spot Captain Landry approaching with the sun rising behind her. I stop to salute her, waiting to see if she is looking for me or passing by. "At ease."

"Yes, Ma'am."

"We are being moved to Belgium along with most of the evacuation hospital. A unit has been over there, setting up our new location. Please help prepare the others to implement standard protocol for transferring patients who we expect to make a full recovery. The others are having arrangements made on their behalf."

The words, "Yes, Ma'am," don't feel as though they are coming out of my mouth. Another wave of shock runs through me like a dry sponge against a brick. Everett was right.

Captain Landry takes a glance around before placing her hand on my back and guiding me several yards away from the tents. "Lizzie, I know how concerned you are for Lieutenant Anderson, but I need you to know my hands are tied this time. He will not be moving to Belgium with us."

All I can do is offer a nod of my head, feeling the drain of emotions slip through my body. The thought of giving up and succumbing, so the struggle will be over, feels easier than continuing. It's a horrible thought to consider, but one that has crossed my mind many times.

"I will alert the others," I say.

"Lizzie, Germany is not a safe place for you. I need you to be aware. We've been kept away from the Nazis in this location, but I'm afraid we won't be facing the same situation once we move."

As if there was more breath to steal from my lungs, I am sure there is not an ounce of oxygen left in my body now. "I will keep my head down and stay away from any hint of trouble, Ma'am."

"I want to keep you safe."

"Thank you, Ma'am."

Once Captain Landry is out of sight, I return to the tent and race to Everett's bedside. "I have some bad news," I tell him, dropping to my knees.

"What is it?" he asks.

"You were correct. I'm not sure where you are being sent, but you aren't coming with the rest of us to Belgium."

Everett struggles to lift his hand and touch the side of my face. "I don't want you to go there."

"I don't have a say in the matter."

He closes his eyes for a moment and opens them, but he locks his stare on the pitch of the tent rather than me. "What if one of us doesn't make it back home?"

It's the first time Everett has verbalized this question that's most likely been ruminating in his brain all this time. With all that we have been through, he has tried to stay positive even when suffering in silence. He did that to keep my spirits up. Even in his battle-scarred state, he's been trying to take care of me.

"Home," I state. I close my eyes for a moment too, recalling the conversation I had with the salesman in the furniture story the day I was foolishly planning out my future, looking at fabrics and colors. "Home is wherever we are together; wherever that may be."

Everett has a pained look upon his face. "I don't want to wonder which of us will be the last one to come home."

"Then don't. It will happen. Life isn't a race, it's just time unfolding the way it's supposed to."

I kiss Everett's lips and do everything possible to hold back the hot tears burning the backs of my eyes. "Everything will be okay."

"You keep saying this," he whispers.

"We have to believe it. It's the only way we'll get through this."

"Lizzie," he mutters.

"What is it?" I trace my fingers around his ear.

"I know you think I don't understand everything, but when I asked you to marry me, I was serious." He takes my hand away from his face and kisses my ring finger. "It's the first thing I want to do when we both get home."

"The very first thing," I promise. "I want nothing more than to spend the rest of our lives—at home together."

Everett quirks a small smile. "That's all I need to get by."

47

MARCH 1945

IF SOMEONE TOLD me seventeen weeks ago, that the worst was yet to come, I'm not sure I would have believed them, but for months on end, we have been within enemy lines, being shot at day and night while doing everything in our power to keep the patients safe. What looks like fireworks at night are flares lighting up the sky with artillery. The organization in Germany is not the same as it was in France. We've moved several times, which has meant transporting patients through battle zones while keeping an eye out for potential attacks. Whenever we find ourselves situated for a short time, it gives us just enough minutes or hours to tally up how much we have lost.

All our men's faces look the same now. The weak, tired, hopeless look in their eyes matches the way I feel inside. We've lost so many, and yet until these past few weeks, we would continue to bring in more casualties, amputate more limbs, patch up missing eyes, and do our best to keep these men alive. But lately, we have noticed less American casualties among our patients. I'm not sure if this is a sign of accomplishment or utter failure.

Captain Landry told us we are coming toward the end of our travels as we approach the southern region of Germany, but it doesn't mean much at this point since we have lost all sense of hopefulness.

The battle is not over, and the damage to the villages we travel through is ongoing and incomprehensible. War was incited and carried out by an enemy with no regard for innocent lives lost or civilians stripped of all they hold dear. Homes of the innocent are in piles of ashes on the ground, and rubble, debris, and soot cover every inch of the cobblestone roads. Families stand helpless in the streets, starving, pale, and frozen with no idea what to think when they see an American passing by.

Swastikas decorate every square foot of these small towns and I can't help but wonder if Hitler knows what his army has done to their own while on their quest to eradicate all Jews and other innocent people who don't meet his standards of perfection. No person with a beating heart could bear witness to these sights without falling apart and call themselves a human. The monster named Hitler has destroyed so much of the world, and here I am standing in the center of his evil. Nazis still march the streets with their fear tactics and weapons as if they have won the battle—the one they are so clearly losing.

"Do you see that, up ahead?" Maggie asks. We're riding in the back of one of our ambulatory vehicles, and from what we know, we're making our way to a city in need of urgent medical care for allied troops, suffering civilians, and some liberated prisoners.

"What are you looking at?" Beverly asks.

Maggie places her hands on the back of my head, tilting my focus to the right. I narrow my eyes to make out what I'm seeing. "Stop the vehicle," I shout, banging on the metal sides.

"What are you doing?" Maggie asks.

"What do you mean? You see what I see, don't you?"

"There are Nazi's pushing along a parade of prisoners, yes, Lizzie. We all see it." Beverly adds.

"We have to help."

Maggie grabs my hand so firmly, I almost yelp. "Are you out of your mind? They will kill you without hesitation. You can't go out there, Lizzie. You can't."

"Where are they taking all of those people?" I realize Maggie doesn't have the answer to my question, but I thought the prisoners are in camps. Now they're walking through the woods, barefoot in nothing more than pajamas. The officer riding in the front of our vehicle approaches the back gate of the vehicle. "What's the problem?"

I point through the thin leafless trees. Some prisoners spot us and stop in their tracks to observe the distraction in what could be their path to safety. "We have to help them," I repeat.

"We don't have the means to go head-to-head with a group of Nazis, nor do the three of you know how to fight."

"Give me a weapon," I demand.

"Ignore her, Sir. She needs more sleep, and she's—" Maggie tries to stop me.

"I have been fighting behind the scenes for years with no sense of accomplishment. At this moment, I feel like I have nothing more to lose and it's an opportunity to attack those who are torturing the innocent souls standing before us."

"No," the officer says without hesitation. "We need you, as a nurse to keep as many of our men breathing as you can. We need you alive, Lieutenant."

Maybe I've had enough. I don't know if Everett is home and safe. I don't know if he's alive or dead. My brothers, God only knows where they are, or if they are okay, and I haven't been able to communicate with Dad in over three months. What if this is my sole purpose right now—the reason I'm on this earth—to free these suffering souls from any more misery?

The hundreds of prisoners continue marching forward in response to the shouts and orders coming from each side of them, and I watch in horror.

Some of those who are marching fall and struggle to stand back up. Others try to help the fallen, taking an immediate beating when caught. And then there are several who are falling behind in the shadows, waiting to take in their last breaths as they gaze up at the sky.

I push my way out of the vehicle past Maggie and the officer. The vehicles in the convoy behind us come to a halt and other troops approach with questions.

"I'm going to help those people over there. They need us," I cry out.

"At least wait until the rest of us are not in sight, Elizabeth,"

Maggie says, grunting with wrath. I don't think I've ever heard her so brazen before now.

"Oh, for God's sake, let's just go help," Beverly says, marching forward.

"If you aren't coming with me, lend me that weapon," I tell the officer. In no way should I be speaking in this manner to anyone with a higher rank than me, but I'm at the end of my rope and I will not stand by and watch a scene from a horror movie play out in front of my eyes after devoting everything we have to put a stop to this nightmare.

"Lieutenants, get back into the vehicle at once," the officer shouts in a demanding voice. His face turns a deep, bitter shade of red, and I know time is of the essence. I spot a weapon in one of the open cubbies within the wagon of the ambulance, and without hesitation, I lunge for the rifle and move past the others who are pleading with me to stop.

"Elizabeth," Maggie shouts. "You're going to get yourself killed."

"Or she can retaliate and avenge the deaths of her people," Beverly shouts. "And maybe save some lives in the process."

I can't believe the words spilling from Beverly's mouth. It's numbing to listen to, but I have to focus on the situation at hand.

My pulse is thrashing in my ears, my lungs feel as though I can't take in enough air, but I am stronger than I have ever been before. Years of living in fear of being a Jewish woman will not stop me from saving as many of these people who have dropped to their knees in the cold, ready to die, or pleading for mercy, as I can.

I figured someone would have pulled us away from the direction we are approaching, but instead, I find our troops behind us, following closely. I stop at the first fallen body, checking for a pulse, but there isn't one.

The anger within me comes to a head. To imagine how long this woman has survived only to die alone in the woods — is inconceivable. I move forward to the next person lying on the frozen earth. Her eyes are open, her skin is gray, and her bones look as though they are caving into the barren cavity of her body. Her chest struggles to rise, then collapses as if gravity doesn't exist. This woman looks like the world is about to fall on top of her, but they have pushed her beyond fear, and she appears to be waiting for the end to spare her more agony. Tears and holes cover her clothes that barely conceal her skeletal form, and I couldn't guess at her age. She has young eyes but looks to have lived beyond a lifetime in Hell. "I'm going to help you," I tell her.

"Gather up the fallen," one of our soldiers gives orders. I'm grateful they decided to help and that I'm not alone in believing these tattered lives deserve a chance to survive. I stop at the first body I come across and carefully lift the woman into my arms, realizing she must not weigh more than sixty pounds. I feel as though I might break her in half if I move the wrong way.

"Thank you," she whimpers.

While following the path out of the woods and back toward the vehicles, the sound of crunching leaves against ice and snow pulls my attention from a direction behind me. I'm careful to lower the woman down against a large rock, then turn on my heels, finding a guard walking toward our direction.

"Halt!" he commands. "Verlasse sie."

From the corner of my eye, I spot Beverly to my right, near a cluster of trees. I hadn't seen her a moment earlier, but she's helping another fallen prisoner. I'm surprised to see her trying to save someone wearing a yellow star sewn to her sleeve, but at the moment, my biggest fear is what she might do with a weapon in her hand.

Beverly stands and holds her hands up to the guard, one hand gripping a pistol she's aiming at the sky. "Don't you have enough prisoners? You must have a heart somewhere deep inside of you. Let us help them," she calls out to the Nazi.

I want to tell her to shut her mouth because it wouldn't take much for this brainwashed guard to respond to her words with gunfire. Beverly must feel a false sense of security as she momentarily takes her eyes off the guard. She leans down toward the fallen prisoner just as the Nazi lifts his pistol, screaming, "Heil Hitler!" at the top of his lungs. The seconds play out as if in slow moving seconds, and I'm frozen while watching Beverly shudder. Her eyes go wide with terror, and I'm not sure where to keep my focus, but she cries out for help, pleading for her life. They are words I never expected to hear from her.

He's going to kill her if I don't do something.

A flashing memory races through my mind from when Dad took me to the shooting range as a young girl. I didn't understand the need for weapons, or why someone would have to kill another to save their life, or someone else's. "I hope you will never need to use a weapon of any kind, but in case you do, I want you to know how to hit your target," he said. I listened to his every word, followed the precise directions, and pulled the trigger. I hit my targets, almost without effort. "I'm impressed by your skills, kiddo. You must take after your old man."

At this moment, I can only pray I wasn't experiencing beginners' luck, and that I do take after Dad.

The guard fires his weapon—the blast echoes between the trees, piercing my ears like knives driving into my head. The sound of a cry howls through the air.

The Nazi engaged first. He had a choice. He made the wrong one.

I release the safety on the pistol in my hand, close my right eye, aim, and pull the trigger. It was Beverly's life or his. The blow knocks me back a foot, but I regain my balance, ready to shoot again if necessary. I hear the thud before I see the damage, finding the Nazi down on his back, clutching his chest.

I feel no remorse for taking his life. I should feel something, but I don't because he was heartless and cold-blooded.

Other soldiers from our convoy race to my side, shouting at me to run. Two of the men scoop up the prisoners, and while I want to listen to their orders this time, I see Beverly lying in a pile of brush, staring back at me with tear-filled eyes. I race to her side and kneel by her head.

She's holding her shoulder, looking whiter than the snow around her body. Blood stains the insides of her fingers, but the location she's holding gives me hope that the bullet only grazed her. "Let me see," I tell her.

"No, just let me die," she says. "It's what I deserve."

"What are you talking about? You do not deserve to die, Beverly, and you will not. Do you hear me?"

"I have no right to your compassion after the way I've treated you."

"Stop talking, Beverly. I don't want to hear you speak that way."

"That Nazi didn't even know I'm Jewish," Beverly groans, "and yet, he still wanted to kill me. I figured if I played the part, as if I weren't Jewish, no one would know—not even you."

The shock of hearing Beverly's words—that she is Jewish has me questioning everything about her. I'm relieved to know I haven't been the only one, but very confused about why she kept it a secret—more than a secret, really. She used it against me. Why did she berate me and treat me so horribly?

"I don't understand, Beverly. Why did you keep that a secret all this time? You seemed so angry at me for being here and putting the rest of you in jeopardy because of my religion."

She sniffles and peers up at me, clutching her shoulder harder. "Because I've been hiding who I am for most of my life. I thought nobody liked Jews, so I was ashamed. When I found out you were Jewish, and proud to be so, I felt angry, but not at you. I was angry at myself, but I took it out on you. Now you saved the life of someone who's been terrible to you and I will never forgive myself. I am so sorry, Elizabeth."

"Beverly, I forgive you, and you are going to survive this hatred right alongside me. And once we're not together anymore, you will still survive, but you should feel proud of who you are."

Tears run down her dirt smudged cheeks, and her eyelids fall heavily as she grits her teeth.

"Beverly," I call out, trying to snap her out of the silence. Her eyelashes bat as if startled, but she's unfocused as she tries to set her gaze on me.

I pull her hand away from her arm, finding the wound to be on the outer layer of skin. "You are going to be fine," I tell her. "It's not a severe wound."

"It's not?" she asks, shivering in my arms.

"No, it's not. I promise. I need help to get this nurse up," I call out. The volume of my voice causes a wave of panic, not knowing how many more Nazis are marching through these woods.

Thankfully, a soldier is behind me within seconds, helping me get her up and over to the truck. Isabel runs out from another ambulance toward us to help with Beverly.

"What in the world happened? Beverly!" she shouts. "Come on, honey, we have room in our vehicle."

"She took a graze just below her shoulder," I tell Isabel.

"I'll take care of her," she says, helping the soldier carry her to the truck.

Within minutes, we are driving much faster than before.

Maggie isn't speaking. She seems taken aback in shock or angered—likely both. Plus, I imagine I'm in trouble for disobeying orders, but I can't say I care at this point.

"Are you injured?" I ask the woman we found in the woods, having only a little space in the truck to examine her.

She places her hand on her stomach and I drape a sheet over her to look at her abdomen. There is a deep hematoma bulging from the area just above her belly button. It's black and purple with a yellow ring around it, but the rest of her looks like a skeleton with a thin layer of tissue like skin covering the protruding bones.

"She's starving," Maggie says, from the other side of the ambulance, tending to another woman. "There is only skin and bones left on this woman too."

"How far from the hospital are we?"

"I don't think we're far," Maggie says.

48

JULY 1945

OVER THE LAST SEVERAL MONTHS, we have cared for tens of thousands of liberated, but displaced civilians, and American and allied military prisoners of war. The malnutrition and diseases were a different battle we had to fight, always trying to beat the clock that threatened to steal their lives. I've heard stories from some other nurses and medics that sound like something you'd read in a fictional horror book. But the stories are true. I have observed wounds unlike any I have seen before, and I've had to accept that the emotional trauma inflicted on these battered souls may be permanent. The empty look in so many eyes, the anger, the longing to die so they wouldn't have to remember what happened, has eaten away at my core. I want to take away their pain and nightmares, but the only way to do that would be to erase their memories. I can't imagine how they will go on after living through this nightmare, but God willing, they will find strength. I've lost count of how many liberated Jews I've treated and for each set of eyes staring back at me, I see a mirroring reflection of myself—a Jewish woman, lucky enough to have been born in the United States which is the only reason I was not sitting beside them in cell blocks, starving, disease-ridden, receiving torture, or facing a slaughtering. I don't understand how people can be so cruel, or how any of us can move on after what we've seen, but we must so we can share what we've learned and pray that it never happens again.

The war seems as though it is coming to an end here, but the scars of those I'm leaving behind will last long after we are gone. The agony these innocent people endured will haunt me forever, but I will always be grateful that I helped them, even if it was in the smallest way.

My heart aches as I approach the end of my time here, but a part of me will remain in these cold, unforgiving woods, wishing I could have done more, but feeling a sense of confidence and honor knowing I did all I could.

My purpose seems clear now—something I pondered most of my life. For everything I've witnessed, and the part of my soul I've lost, I learned firsthand, after being painfully close to something I knew nothing about, that there's no room in this world for intolerance or hatred. Nobody wins when there is a war. We're all one, and no matter how trying life can be, fighting is never the answer, but being willing to lend a hand to help one another, is. That's what I needed to do on my journey to self-fulfillment. I succeeded.

Now, we're going home. Home feels like it has too many meanings to comprehend. I wasn't sure I'd make it to this day. As I prepare to travel back to my home, I hope to instill a sense of pride and teach others about the difference one person's hands can make.

49

JULY 1945

US SOIL. Did I walk away from a world on pause, or did three years of my life slip by without me knowing?

During my flights back to the states, I had more time on my hands than I would have liked, and in the quiet moments when people were napping, I lied awake, pondering how I managed to walk through flying bullets without one taking me down. I don't understand why, even though I may be a little ragged around the edges, I'm in perfect physical condition while other lives are being mourned. Why is one life chosen over another? It's a question I don't think I will ever have an answer to.

I wonder if I will face a punishment for my actions that some are calling heroic. I shot a man—killed him, but I saved thousands. Will my conduct shift the balance of Everett's future? It's a foolish way to look at life, but when I think back to every stop along the way over the last three years, I question if it was a lesson in the form of a nightmare. It seems unthinkable as I look back on it—something a mind could never conjure, yet it's branded into the faint lines on my forehead and in the corners of my weak smile while I try to comprehend that I'm going home.

I don't know who is aware of my homecoming because there wasn't enough time between finding out I was heading back to the states and sending a letter to let Dad know I'm on my way. I haven't hugged him in three years. I haven't seen James, and

Lewis—I don't know where he is, or if he is still okay. Our last hug was when he told me Everett was still alive. I fear going home to a barren world resembling the crumbling ash-covered existence I left behind.

Still, I straighten my cap and collar and walk eloquently out of the airport terminal. As if someone silenced the sound of revolving life during the time I was gone, it restarts with a scratch on a record, growing in volume—in the form of conversation, laughter, and reminiscing cheers. I search through the crowd for a familiar face without knowing what to expect.

My steps feel long and drawn out as I part my way through groups of people and a world I'm about to rejoin, but when I see his face, a sense of warmth and comfort fills every fiber in my body.

This moment reminds me of the time I had the stomach bug in grade school, and the teacher sent me to the nurse's office to wait for someone to come pick me up. I had never felt so sick, and I was scared, counting down the minutes until someone would come tell me I would be okay. I wasn't expecting to see Dad walk into the school that day. Mom was usually the one who would have to come to my rescue if I needed to go home early. But there he was, sharp as ever in his uniform, bearing a smile that made me forget about the discomfort traveling through my body. I cried at the sight of him for reasons I still don't understand. I just needed him, as a little girl—I needed my dad to make me all better. The moment his arms were around me and he placed a kiss on the top of my head, I knew I was okay.

My chin quivers as I see the man walking toward his little girl with a smile full of pride and his arms open just for me. Neither of us can speak. Again, words aren't necessary because his embrace is everything the little girl in me needs right now. For the first time in years, I know I'm going to be okay. His love says it all.

It's minutes before each of us can compose ourselves enough to speak. "I went to bed so many nights wondering if I had taught you well enough to survive in a war that I never expected you to be a part of. It was my job to keep you safe, and I didn't know if I failed you and your mother, but when news broke from other commanding officers of your bravery and accomplishments, I realized you didn't need me to guide you anymore because you have an inner strength beyond anything your mother or I ever had. Your determination, courage, and commitment has outshone us all, Elizabeth. The word pride does not begin to explain what I feel for you, my daughter."

I nod because I am at a loss for words. I don't know where to start, I suppose. Dad takes my duffle bag in one arm and takes my hand with the other. "I missed you so much, Dad," I mutter.

"Oh, sweetheart, a girl will always love her father, but she will never know how much more he loves her. Each day you weren't here, felt like a decade."

"Lewis and James?" I ask.

"They are home and well, eagerly waiting for me to bring you home. They wanted to come with me, but I asked them for this time alone with you. I hope that's okay."

I press my cheek against his arm and take in a sigh of relief. "Of course, it is." I take a minute to find the courage to ask a question haunting every part of me. "Dad—"

It seems that's all I can manage to say when he interrupts whatever he thinks I was going to ask. "It's been a while since I've heard anything. I know they sent Everett home so his father could care for him, but I haven't heard an update as of late. However, I called his father's house to let him know you were on your way home, but there was no answer. I also had a telegram delivered to his house, but honestly, I'm not sure of his current condition. I'm sorry, Elizabeth. I wish I had something better to tell you."

The hollowness in my chest reminds me of my missing heart, the one I left with him when we separated in Belgium. It's been months and if his condition worsened after our last goodbye, he may not know who I am at all now. It's a thought I've dreaded, but one I accept as a possible reality.

"Audrey is impatiently waiting at our house for you, as well. She has someone she'd like you to meet, but if she knows I told you this, I might be in a lot of trouble, so you have to act surprised, okay?"

Audrey and I wrote to each other several times while we were away, but we weren't able to stay in contact as much as I hoped. She also enlisted in the Army Nurse Corps, and her deployment and unit remained on ship from what I understand. I believe she returned home only recently.

"I guess I'm the last one home, huh?"

"We were hoping you'd be back a few months ago, but your unit was needed for good reason." All along, I thought we were losing more and more every day we spent over there.

"Is there anything else I should know about before I step back into this life I left behind?"

"Yes," Dad says. "There is something you need to know."

"Okay, I'm ready."

I watch the surrounding civilians, moving about the airport seeking their next destination. Street clothes are more common than my uniform, and so many people have flowered leis dangling from their necks. Children are laughing and chasing each other in circles around their parents, and the fresh scent of fruit fills the air. I forgot what it felt like to be here.

"When you return home from battle, no matter what your position, or your responsibilities were, or what it forced you to do, think, and see—it changes you—inside. Some people think you've become hardened, and others pity what you experienced. And then there's the part that you feel. When you peer into a mirror, you may not recognize yourself as the same person you used to be. You may see a look of pain riddled throughout your eyes, or the face of a fading soul reaching out for help. The moments in combat are the memories that scar you deeply. They change who you are, who you were, and who you will be, but if there is anything I have learned over the years, it's this: for every anguished thought that enters your mind, replace it with the memory of something good you did. You saved so many people, Elizabeth, and that's what you should focus on."

"I'm fine, Dad, really."

"You're going to say that. You're going to convince yourself you're okay, but there are going to be moments when you aren't, and I need you to know that I am here to listen, and I will always be that person in your life no matter what. I understand you, what you've been through, and what you will continue to go through. You never have to feel like you're alone."

I want to respond with a quick thank you and move on, but I

allow the words to penetrate, knowing he's right. Over the last day, I lost track of how many spiraling thoughts spun through my head like a tornado, distracting me, exhausting me, and adding confusion to my overwhelmed mind.

"You know, now that I've seen the other side, you should know you can always talk to me too," I tell Dad.

"That's what best friends do for each other, kiddo. You will always be my little girl, but we share something unique now too."

"James and Lewis, as well," I add.

We step out of the airport into the most exquisite Hawaiian glow and I lift my face to the sky to inhale all the sweet aromas I have missed. "It's good to be home."

"Elizabeth," Dad says, tugging my hand so I stop walking. "I know how you feel about feeling equal to your brothers. You have always made it a point to prove your sense of worth to me and them, but there is a difference between you three, and I think it's important you understand."

"What's the difference?" I shrug with a small laugh.

"They trained for combat, Elizabeth. You trained to heal and save the lives of our own. Maybe you don't think I'm aware of what you accomplished a couple months back, but the news did not come quietly here at home. You stood up to a fear greater than any one of us could comprehend, and without hesitation, saved over twelve dying prisoners from what is being called 'a death march.' Your bravery was unfathomable, and while I know you are humble and will probably never mention the subject, what you did will forever make me proud of the woman I raised."

Am I receiving praise for the death I caused, or the lives I saved? It's a question I continue to ask myself. That day in the woods will always haunt me because I had to take a life to save one. The world shouldn't be so ugly that one life has to be chosen over another.

I try to press my lips into a smile, but it hurts too much. Thankfully, Dad understands the look on my face. Rather than focus on what I'm being recognized for, I find our shadows along the curb, recalling a time when mine was so small compared to his. But now, they are nearly identical; I might be shorter and more slender, but our posture, stature, and form of stride are the same.

We are equal.

Dad allows me what I need; quiet moments during the car ride home, with the windows open. I take in the view of the passing seascape, the sun, and clouds in all their glorious buoyancy within the Hawaiian sky. I watch a plane skim the top of a cloud and feel the need to wave, but instead, I smile, wondering if it's just another plane, or possibly a sign I need to see.

As we turn the corner onto our street, I hold my breath, wondering if Everett's car will be along the curb. Dad isn't the type to cause me pain just for the sake of a surprise. I should have assumed he wasn't making up a story when he said he hasn't heard from him.

"Whose car is that?" I ask, hoping beyond hope.

"I'll let your brother tell you," Dad says.

"What is it?"

"I've already said too much, telling you that Audrey has news. Just go on in and find out for yourself. I'll get your bags."

The house smells just how I left it. Everything is clean, not a crooked picture frame in sight. I can't say I imagined the house would look so neat but it's comforting to come home to.

I appreciate that no one lunges at me as I walk in the door. Instead, warm hugs, kisses on the head, and the feeling of so much love welcomes me home. James and Lewis each want to show their affection more than the other, and I feel them elbowing each other behind my back.

"You already got to see her once. It's my turn," James says, squeezing me within his arms as he lifts me up and spins me in a circle before placing me down in front of a familiar face.

"Lokelani," I greet her. "You're still here—with James?" I take a moment to comprehend the meaning, and the fact that she's here in my house almost four years after I saw her that one time.

She's also pregnant and there's a ring on her finger. I spin around, looking for James's expression, and I find one more perfect than I could ever wish for him. He's beaming.

"I wanted to wait for you, kiddo."

"Well, to be fair, I was gone a long time," I offer as a good reason not to wait for me.

"We eloped when I returned home six months ago. It was small and just the two of us. You know I don't like to make a big deal out of anything."

"Of course," I tell him. Though it pains me to think I missed out on something big in James's life, I can't blame him for taking the first opportunity he had to make his life feel normal and happy after this war.

"I'm the same way," Lokelani says. "Also, I hope you don't mind that I helped around here a bit while you were overseas. Your father and brothers were helpless it seemed. Then, with their staggering deployments, I couldn't help myself. I knew you would want your family cared for. I remember you told me it was your biggest concern before leaving."

My gaze falls to my fidgeting fingers as I silently thank mom for sending all of us who we needed when we needed them. Although Lewis is alone, he isn't the type to need another person to make him happy. He is content with being around happiness, just like Mom was.

I offer Lokelani a gentle hug, careful not to squish her growing belly. "How far along are you?" I ask.

"Twenty-two weeks," she says, beaming with a smile from ear to ear.

"I can't wait to meet my niece or nephew. What a wonderful surprise to come home to." I turn in the last direction I haven't paid attention to yet. "And you, Miss, what do you have to say for yourself?"

Audrey all but nearly pummels me to the ground as she slams into me with a force full of a thousand hugs saved up over the few years. "I'm so thankful we're both alive and here. I'm so thankful, Lizzie. These have been the longest years of my life, and I can't believe we're together in the same room, finally."

"Yeah, yeah, I missed you too, but um, who's the charming fella standing behind you?"

Audrey's cheeks burn red as she dances around in a little circle to grab the gentleman by the arm. "Lizzie, this is Pierre

Lucas. We met when my unit docked off the coast of Monaco. He was delivering goods to our crew, and well—"

"Ooh-la-la," I gush with the worst French accent I can muster. "Well, what is it?" Excitement fills my chest for the first time in a very long while.

"I guess love at first sight is a real thing," she says, shrugging her shoulders against her shy smile.

Pierre reaches out for my hand. "Bonjour, Mademoiselle. Is a pleasure to ah—make your acquaintance."

"Excuse me," I say, pulling my hand from Pierre's. "What is that gorgeous, sparkling rock on your hand?"

"Lizzie, Pierre asked me to marry him." I wring my arms around Audrey's neck squeezing her with all my might, feeling an abundance of happiness for my closest friend.

Then, a brick falls into the pit of my stomach as I witness the warm affectionate smile grow along Pierre's cheeks as he watches our shared excitement.

"Gosh, I am blown away by all of this," I tell them. "This is— well this is so swell. I can't believe all that I have been missing out on. Will you excuse me for a moment? I just need to use the restroom to powder my nose."

I try to take slow breaths, in and out, telling myself everything is okay, and sometimes life works out in funny ways, but it isn't always full of big band swing music and long days by the shore. Sometimes we must put ourselves aside and just show happiness for others, which I am. I am so glad for all of them and their joy.

The moment I close the bathroom door, I slide down against the wood molding until I reach the glossy tiles. Tears flow freely like a burst pipe that had been holding in way too much for far too long. I cry until my lungs burn, my head aches, and my chest sinks in toward my back. I don't know if this is the way I will always be, a cheery face with a fake smile to hide the truth inside, or if I'm going to adjust and find my place here again. I suppose it's something I won't know until life unfolds one day at a time.

* * *

My family allowed me to sit on the bathroom floor for three straight hours until there was a knock. We only have one bathroom, and I should have picked a better place to fall apart. I open the door, finding the house empty except for Dad and Lewis.

"Let's listen to some music and take it easy," Lewis says as Dad pulls me out of the bathroom to switch places with me.

50

JULY 1945

My HAND TREMBLES as I attempt to form a straight line along the curves of my lips with the red, waxy crayon that makes my eyes glow like the color of hazelnuts. It's taken me a few days to get my bearings and put away all my belongings, and I feel better except for missing the leading male actor of what feels like a movie that lasted far too long.

I've tried to call Everett several times over the last few days but there hasn't been an answer at his father's house, or at least the number Dad had gotten for his father's house. I've gone as far as contacting his former captain to see if he had a different way to reach him, but he said he would get back to me if he could find out anything regarding his whereabouts. I hate that the answer must always be patience because I have run out of whatever that is supposed to mean.

"Are you ready?" Dad asks, poking his head in through my open bedroom door.

"I think so." I wish Maggie or Isabel were here to join me. Heck, I might even settle for Beverly now that she's seen 'the light' as she described after being stitched up. The commencement speech a commander is giving today has something to do with the 2nd evacuation hospital, so it doesn't feel right attending without my unit. We've all gone back to our families, though. At least Audrey will be there standing next to me as an Army nurse, too.

Lewis and Dad are both in their dress greens, and in their natural state of being quiet and reserved as they wait for me to walk out the door first. "Even after being in the Army for three years, it still feels like you two, or three, when James is here, follow me around like personal guards. Does it ever get old?" I ask.

"Yes," Lewis says with a snicker.

"Never," Dad follows.

Lewis opens the passenger side door for me to slide in and bows his head to duck into the backseat. There was a time when I could never claim a seat in the front because of the sheer amount of bickering between James and Lewis. Of course, they would both squeeze in and there was no point in trying to find a place up there with them. The back seat has always been a nice quiet place to stare out the window. I wouldn't mind it much now either, but I suppose we're all a bit old for arguing over who sits where.

The ride is short, and the rows of cars are endless when we arrive. "I didn't realize this was such a big commencement ceremony today. Is this only our base?"

"It is, but we've accomplished a lot over the last few years, and it's important to recognize our efforts," Dad says.

I'm able to find Audrey rather quickly, giving me a friend to stand with as we melt in our uniforms underneath the unforgiving sun.

Speeches are never short with the military, but they are always enlightening. Today, though, I'm having trouble focusing on much else other than finding a way to track Everett down. There must be more contact information for him somewhere.

"We have several medals we would like to award today. The efforts over the last four years have been anything but easy, especially after rebounding from such a horrific catastrophe right here in our backyards. On behalf of the United States Army and Navy, we are deeply grateful for every one of you who have served and dedicated yourselves to our country."

The list of names is long, and my legs threaten to fall asleep. I feel the need to rest my head on Audrey's shoulder, but I know well it will cause us both to fall into a fit of laughter that will get us in trouble. "Has it always been this hot here?" I whisper.

"Yes," she mutters in response. "Shh."

"There is one medal we are awarding here on our base for an outstanding accomplishment on the battlefield and here at home. This person has gone above and beyond their call of duty to save innocent beings from the cruelties of war. Never, have we given out this achievement award, and I am privileged to present one out of the twenty-one of these medals that we are handing out across the country. Captain, if you would please do the honors."

A plane whizzes through the sky, distracting me from the recognition speech, but Audrey pinches my underarm to bring me back to the moment. "Ouch," I shout through a quiet whisper.

"This United States Army nurse deserves more than a medal for her heroic actions, but it is my honor to present First Lieutenant Elizabeth Salzburg with this Bronze Star Medal."

I squint toward the podium, shocked at hearing my name called, and telling myself to move, but also taking a second to inspect the hands holding the medal.

My legs move of their own accord, one foot in front of the other, as I wish on every cloud in the sky that I'm not hallucinating from dehydration beneath this hot sun. When I'm only a few feet away, I cup my gloved hands around my mouth and pause in place because even though I'm melting, I'm frozen. I can't go any further. I can't endure another moment of hope if it's not real.

"Before I present you with this medal, I would like to ask you a question, if you wouldn't mind … doll-face?"

He steps down from the platform, walking with slow, long strides toward me like a man in armor rather than a man in uniform. With a struggle, he kneels and holds out the medal in the palm of his white glove. Next to the medal is a ring.

"Elizabeth Salzburg, not only have you saved my life in more ways than a man should ever have to be saved, but you have taught me the true meaning of home and offered me a chance to feel undying love and devotion. You gave me hope, a reason to keep going, and a sense of normal when all I knew was turmoil and heartache. For you, I kept my head up day after day and refused to succumb to the hands pulling me away from a life, I knew I wanted and needed. I don't want to be apart from you again, and I want to spend every minute of the rest of my life making you as proud of me as I am of you. So please, sweetheart, do me this honor, and marry me?"

I fall to my knees because the rush of emotions is too much to bear. Everett is home. He's walking, speaking, and alive. The man I love more than anything in this world is alive, and he wants to be with me. I feel undeserving of everything in his hands and all that he is offering but after being selfless for so long, I might be okay with this one selfish act. I throw my arms around him, knocking him off his knee while acting completely and utterly inappropriate for a military celebration, but I don't hear a peep. I don't see another soul. It's just him and me, and I'm kissing the lips I feared I would never get to touch again.

"I want to see all the world's wonders with you and even fly you up through those clouds we adore. Will you marry me?" Everett asks again, mumbling against my lips.

"Yes," I say, gasping for air while I try to speak. "Yes, Everett, yes—you're alive. You're alive. Yes, I'll marry you."

"You're probably killing the poor guy, Elizabeth," Dad says from behind me, pulling me off Everett. Dad reaches down to help him up to his feet, and I watch the struggle he endures, but all I see is the mountain he has climbed and conquered. "I want you two to have a long happy life together. So please, be careful with my future son-in-law, will you?"

Dad wraps his arms around us both and kisses my forehead. "You knew he was here?" I ask Dad.

"No, not until last night. That's why I left right after dinner. Everett made his way home and wanted to make sure he requested my permission before asking for your hand today."

"I received your Dad's telegram, the phone calls from my former Colonel, and my current captain," Everett says, reaching out to pinch my cheek.

Lewis makes his way over and places his hand down on Everett's shoulder. "Congratulations to the both of you," he says.

"Lewis, I could never thank you enough for what you did back there in France." Everett takes in a shaky breath and stares off into the distance. "I don't know how you knew—"

Dad slaps his hands down on my shoulders. "It was because of this chatterbox here who wanted to break every communication regulation the military has ever put into place. But thank God, my little girl knows how to talk as much as she does because she was cautious, yet precise on what she thought might have happened to you and the others. We tried to get to you sooner, but it was hard to track down your unit."

Everett reaches for my necklace and places it on the outside of my collar. "You will never need to hide this beautiful star again."

"I'm so proud of you for receiving this medal, Elizabeth," Dad says. "Never in my wildest dreams did I think you could achieve something so significant in a day when women have had to prove they are just as strong, if not stronger than the men on the battlefield—what an honor for our family."

"May I?" Everett asks.

"Yes, please," I respond, feeling fireworks explode through the inside of my chest as he secures the medal, and then reaches for my hand. He slips my glove off, one finger at a time, and then slides the ring down into place. "Thank you for always being the sun in my sky; a map that led me to the place I belong—my home."

51

CURRENT DAY - OCTOBER 2018

I'M SEATED at the head of an oversized picnic table with so many pairs of eyes staring at me with what I can only describe as love, but something is amiss.

All these faces—have I missed time, or just forgotten?

A brilliant light appears to my side and I search for the source, finding glowing candles flickering on top of a round vanilla frosted cake. Leah is holding the pastry, walking with slow steps as she approaches the open space at the table where she sets the cake down. "We're going to sing now, okay, Mom?" she asks.

"Yeah, Gran, are you ready?" Makena echoes Leah—the two sounding almost identical when hearing them together.

What a sweet gesture this is, but my mind is foggy, I suppose. I glance around, searching for Everett but he isn't here. Neither is Dad, Lewis, or James. Why aren't any of them here? "Well, sure, that would be lovely, but whom are you singing too?"

"It's Dad's birthday," Carter reminds me again. *Dad's birthday. Everett is their father, of course, I know this. I must have known today is his birthday.*

"Yes, I know, but your father, he isn't here, am I correct?" I ask, watching the wax drip down the sides of the candles onto the sparkling whipped frosting.

"Sure he is, Gran," Makena says. "He's home, just like you always say." Makena points up toward the dark clouds and my heart sinks to the bottom of my stomach. He's home, but I am not. It shouldn't be this way. It was never meant to be like this.

My eyes fall to the dessert plate set down in front of me as I catch the reflection of my eyes through my glass of water. "Well, then, I suppose it might be time I finally go home too. Lewis and James, and my father—they must all be wondering where I am."

"Mom, what are you talking about?" Leah asks, placing her hand on my shoulder.

I glance down the length of the table at Daniel who I recall sharing much of my story with today. The look on his face tells me he understands what I mean, but I'm not sure such a powerful explanation would go over too well for the others tonight. "Oh, I don't know. I'm just a chatty old lady, I guess," I say, waving the questions away. "Makena, do you know where the journal is—the one you gave me recently?"

I find Makena's eyes, watching a downcast expression match the slump in her shoulders. "Gran, I didn't give that journal to you. Papa did, when you were just a girl, remember? It's full of your memories."

"Everett gave this to me. My memories?" I question. "I thought the book was for me to keep track of reminders."

"Mom, you have, for most of your life. We make sure you have the journal in case you want to remember anything you might have forgotten," Leah explains while handing me the leather-bound book.

I flip through the pages to the back cover, finding a yellowed envelope.

I trace my fingers across the soft paper with my name written in all capital letters. Beneath, are the words "Just in case—"

"What is that, Gran?" Makena asks.

My memories are in pieces sometimes, but this envelope—I know what is inside.

I lift the envelope, feeling something fall to my lap.

It takes me a moment to glance down because I know what fell. This time, it has fallen face down and the words I have refused to read are staring back at me.

Doll-face,

This photograph isn't just a portrait of me—it's the person I became because of you. When you see the smile on my face, remember it's there only for you.

I flip the photograph over, instantly going back in time when we were young and carefree, laughing and running blissfully along the shore. That smile. It was one in a million.

"Oh, that's papa," Makena says, easing it from my hand. "Wow, he was a good-looking guy, huh?"

"Only the most stunning man in Hollywood during the 1930s, but I believe my bragging rights ran out quite a while ago," I joke.

While the others are fawning over the photo, I tend to the envelope, slipping out the piece of paper I could never get myself to read. Was dying of old age worthy of reading his "just in case I die before you" letter?

I suppose it won't matter for much longer, so I unfold the paper and find more of his beloved handwriting:

My Dearest Elizabeth,

I apologize for the formality of this letter, but if you're reading this, it means I'm gone, and I assume there isn't a proper nickname to soften these words.

I'm so grateful for the time we've shared, even in the sparse moments we've stolen together here in the United Kingdom.

I know neither of us know what tomorrow holds, but I fear the worst in our current situation, and I need you to know what my intentions are in case I'm not able to tell you myself.

Elizabeth Hope Salzberg, I planned to ask you to marry me, have babies together, and make a large family that would fill our hearts with more joy than we could even imagine. I would never let you give up your endeavors, and I would be an equal partner, happy to share our life together, side by side.

We would go to Paris, Rome, Greece, Switzerland, Fiji, the Caribbean Islands, and yes, through the clouds too—all your adventurous longings would become a reality. Your spark for life, sparked my life, and I wish I could have seen the world with you and experienced the best of what should have come for us. But I suppose I must have fulfilled my purpose in other unexpected ways. Please, for me, go on your adventures, live like you own the world, and be the person you dream of becoming. And always remember that, no matter where you end up, I'll be watching over you to make sure you find your purpose.

I love you more than I've loved anyone or anything in my life. I'm sorry I had to go so soon.

Someday, after you have lived a long, full life and you are ready to come home, I'll be waiting for you in the clouds, riding on top of that crazy flying elephant.

I love you, Lizzie.

Always and forever,

Everett

You gave me all of that and more, Everett. You made all my dreams come true. Every single one.

My heart aches with a pain I haven't felt in longer than I can remember, which I'm thankful for now. I wish I knew how long I've been living this way, or how many years I've gone without finding my way home—the one I belong to with Everett. But I realize my purpose is sitting at this table because it was something we accomplished together.

Yet, I'm still here. Why?

"I shouldn't still be here, should I?" I ask aloud. My question is another cause for concern judging by the multiple sets of wide eyes and fallen jaws. "I'm sorry if I'm upsetting any of you. It's just—there's something next, something unknown, another adventure that's waiting for me."

No one says much, but I hear a low rumble of mutters along both sides of the table. "We don't have to do this right now, Mom," Carter says.

I look at my son, a stunning replica of Everett. How could I not see it before? "You look just like your father," I tell him.

"You've always said this," Carter says, smirking in the same way Everett did. "And Leah looks like you, and so does Makena, Mom. We have some strong genes in this family."

The more I look around, the more familiar everyone's features look. "So, when I leave to go home, part of me will still be here, right?"

"You shouldn't talk this way," Leah says. "But of course, you will always be with us no matter where you are, Mom."

"I miss them all so much, especially your father. Maybe this is the reason my memory doesn't want to work anymore. It's probably a blessing. I suppose there isn't anything easy about being the last one left."

"You always told us Dad said the last one home would have to be the strongest. Neither of you wanted to go first, but if you recall what he said the day, he—went home?" Leah asks, a hitch catching in her throat, "He told you, 'I always knew you were the strongest of us all.'"

I close my eyes and recall holding Everett's hand. His dazzling smile made one more appearance just before he said:

"I'll be home waiting for you, but take your time, doll. Take your time."

Those words filled his last breath, and I know I didn't want to spend a minute without him. The pain was insufferable, but since then, whenever that was, I've been staring aimlessly into the sky in search of my love, wondering why he isn't by my side. Maybe, I've wanted to forget the rest just so I could hold on to him.

"Mom," Leah says, her voice full of concern.

"I remember what he said that day," I say. "How could I forget?"

I push myself up to my feet and take a few steps over to the white fence settled beneath the starry night sky. As I glance up toward the clouds highlighted by the moon's glow, I blow a kiss to my sweetheart and whisper, "Happy birthday, darling. I'm coming home to you now."

REFERENCES

Frank Sinatra and Frank Sinatra and Tommy Dorsey, *"I'll Never Smile Again;"* Artie Shaw, Public domain, via Wikimedia Commons

ALSO BY SHARI J. RYAN

www.sharijryan.com

The Last Words Series
Last Words
The Other Blue Sky
Unspoken Words

The Heart Series
A Heart of Time
A Missing Heart
A Change of Heart

The Barrel House Series
Bourbon Love Notes
Bourbon on the Rocks
Bourbon Nights
Bourbon Fireball

Standalone Novels:
Fall to Pieces
Shattered Stars
Ravel
Raine's Haven

ABOUT THE AUTHOR

Shari J. Ryan is a *USA Today* Bestselling Author of Contemporary Romance and Women's Fiction. Shari was once told she tends to exaggerate often and sometimes talks too much, which would make a great foundation for fictional books. Four years later, Shari has written thirteen novels that often leave readers either in tears from laughing, or crying.

With her loud Boston girl attitude, Shari isn't shy about her love for writing or the publishing industry. Along with writing several International bestsellers, Shari has split her time between writing and her longstanding passion for graphic design. In 2014, she started an indie-publishing resource company, MadHat Books, to help fellow authors with their book cover designs, as well as assistance in the self-publishing process.

While Shari may not find many hours to sleep, she still manages to make time for her family. She is a devoted wife to a great guy, and a mother to two little boys who remind her daily why she was put on this earth.

For more information:

Web:
www.sharijryan.com
Email:
shari@sharijryan.com
Facebook:
/authorsharijryan
Twitter:
@sharijryan
Twitter:

@authorsharijryan

Make sure you join Shari's Reader Group at:
facebook.com/sharijryanvipreaders

Sign up for Shari's newsletter:
Sharijryan.com/subscribe

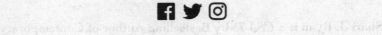

ACKNOWLEDGMENTS

This book took many months to research and hundreds of hours of time. My family has continuously supported by dreams and passion for writing, giving me understanding and space when needed so I can transport myself into another time, and into different pairs of shoes so I can live through my story. I couldn't have gotten to where I am today without you.

Josh, my always and forever. Our hours of endless conversations about fictional characters and worlds mean more to me than you could ever know. Thank you for always lifting me up higher to reach my goals.

Bryce and Brayden, my two sons who make me so proud to be your mother. Your desire to read my stories and know about all my characters helps me fall asleep with a smile at night.

Mom, thank you for spending endless days and nights scouring every words of my book to help me make the story the best it could be. Only one person knows my mind better than me and I'm thankful you have the patience to and desire to step inside of my stories with me.

Dad, thank you for calling me every single day to ask how my story is coming along and for taking an interest in what I love. Knowing you talking about my accomplishments to friends and share my books with anyone who will listen, means the world to me.

Mark and Ev, no one ever asked or told you to love and support me as much as you do. I couldn't be more grateful to have two loving step parents in my life who feel as though you have always been by my side. I feel richer having so much more love in my family thanks to the both of you.

Lori, you are still my #1, my backbone, my sounding board, and best friend. I am lucky to have the best sister to ever exist. I love you!

Heather, Tracey, and Emily, - My Alpha Readers - Thank you isn't enough for the time you spend helping me with my books on a regular basis. Your honesty and encouragement boost my motivation like I can't explain.

Erin, LaTonya, Gab, Elaine, and Lin - Thank you for being the most incredible beta readers. Receiving your feedback gave me the confidence to polish up the story and even take it up a notch. I'm grateful for the time you spent helping me with this book.

Linda - As always, thank you for keeping me sane when I'm about to fall off my chair or crash my head into my keyboard late at night. Not only are you the best of the best when it comes to PR & Marketing, but you are a friend I could never live without.

Freesia - Fate brought us together. I'm sure of it. You have brought so much peace and enlightenment to my life, and straightened my messy artist life out. It didn't take long to know you were more than just someone who could help me along the way. We were clearly meant to be friends too.